SIBO

Foods, Supplements & Medicinal Plants

Isabel M. Rivero

COPYRIGHT & CREDITS

SIBO. Foods, Supplements & Medicinal Plants.
Copyright ©2024 *by* Isabel M. Rivero
All rights reserved

Cover design: Valeria Veretennikova
Photographs by Mareefe and Buntysmum via Pixabay

This book provides general information and is not a substitute for professional medical advice. Neither the publisher nor the author shall be held liable for any damages of any kind arising from the use of this content. Readers assume full responsibility for their decisions, actions, and outcomes.

This book is intended as a reference only and should never be used as a medical manual. Its purpose is to help readers make informed decisions about their health. It is not intended to replace any treatment prescribed by a doctor.

To everyone living with SIBO each day,
who face misunderstanding and the many challenges this condition brings.
This book is for you—
for those who have cultivated patience, even on the most difficult days,
who seek answers when uncertainty feels overwhelming,
and who continue to hold on to hope for healing and a vibrant, fulfilling life.
I wrote it from the depths of my heart, with your well-being in mind and
with respect for every hard moment you've endured.
My hope is that within these pages, you'll find tools, relief, and, above all,
understanding.
Always remember, you are not alone. Your journey matters, your efforts
have purpose, and your health is of infinite value.
With all my love and deepest respect,

Isabel

Prologue: A Guide to Wellness

Dear Readers,

Welcome to this journey toward better health! Since I began sharing my knowledge and experience, my primary motivation has been to make a positive contribution to your lives. That's why, through these pages, I aim to offer valuable information and practical resources that can genuinely help you feel better.

In this book, every piece of advice and remedy has been thoughtfully chosen for its proven effectiveness and practicality in everyday life. You will discover not only medicinal plants, supplements, and accessible foods but also detailed medical insights into this health concern, along with additional tips and answers to the most frequently asked questions–providing you with a practical, comprehensive, and trustworthy guide.

My goal is for this work to be your valuable and practical companion–a resource where you can find tangible tools to support you on your journey toward a healthier, more fulfilling life. Knowing that this work has a positive impact brings me great joy and motivates me to keep going. While writing requires effort, time, and perseverance, the knowledge that my books make a meaningful difference in your lives is my greatest reward.

Because your experiences are my greatest source of inspiration, I would love for you to write to me and share your progress. Feel free to share your progress by writing directly to me at **isabelmriveror@gmail.com**. Your stories inspire me and truly make my efforts worthwhile.

I sincerely hope this practical guide becomes your indispensable pillar on your journey to better health and well-being. Thank you for allowing me to be part of your life.

With love,

Isabel

INTRODUCTION

On our journey toward optimal health, it's essential to understand that no "miracle" remedy–whether it's a medication, herb, supplement, or food–can fully address an illness on its own. Similarly, focusing solely on alleviating symptoms without addressing the underlying "cause" increases the risk of relapse. Treating the root of the problem, however, gradually reduces symptoms and promotes true and lasting recovery.

You may have noticed that, at times, medications don't work as expected. This happens because regaining health requires a holistic treatment approach that addresses the actual cause of the problem at its root. In addition to effective treatments, this approach should include changes in diet, sleep quality, stress management, and overall lifestyle habits.

With this book, we will explore a holistic approach to health. In the first chapter, you'll find key information to help you understand the main causes of this disease, along with its symptoms, types, warning signs, common complications, helpful advice, and the essential medical tests needed for an accurate diagnosis. In the following chapters, we'll dive into strategies to support recovery, including dietary guidance, daily menus, and natural approaches such as supplements and herbal remedies for gradual improvement.

While you can independently choose your preferred remedies, the chapter "**Suggested Practical Plan**" will serve as your primary guide. This section offers a comprehensive approach, addressing all essential aspects of recovery. From there, you'll be directed to other chapters and can apply the recommendations best suited to your unique situation.

It's important to emphasize that the benefits of the recommendations provided in this book are grounded in scientific evidence, rather than personal opinions. At the end, you'll find references and studies supporting each remedy, ensuring you feel confident and secure when applying them.

SIBO

SIBO, or Small Intestinal Bacterial Overgrowth, may feel overwhelming at first, but gaining clarity about how it affects your digestive system can make managing it much more approachable. To put it simply, the small intestine, designed to effectively digest and absorb nutrients, naturally contains only a small number of bacteria. However, when bacteria that normally reside in the colon migrate into the small intestine and start multiplying excessively, they upset the delicate balance, interfering with normal functions and unleashing a chain reaction of discomfort and troublesome symptoms.

One of the biggest challenges with SIBO is that these overgrown bacteria directly compete with your body for nutrients from the food you eat. Instead of nourishing and energizing your body, these nutrients are consumed by the bacteria, which ferment them and produce gases like hydrogen and methane. This process often leads to noticeable issues like bloating, gas, abdominal cramps, and discomfort–most commonly after eating. For many people, these symptoms disrupt not just digestion but their overall sense of well-being, making daily life feel more exhausting and challenging.

But it doesn't stop there. The activity of these bacteria also compromises the integrity of the intestinal lining–a vital barrier that's meant to let nutrients in while keeping harmful substances out. With SIBO, this lining weakens, becoming more permeable, a condition often called "leaky gut." This allows particles that don't belong in the bloodstream to pass through, triggering systemic inflammation and causing additional symptoms like fatigue, joint pain, or a lingering sense of feeling unwell.

This ongoing cycle of inflammation and damage to the intestinal lining disrupts proper digestion and hinders the absorption of key nutrients. Deficiencies in essential vitamins, minerals like iron and calcium, or even critical fatty acids can arise, leading to noticeable challenges such as low energy, hair thinning, weakened immunity, unintentional weight loss, or a general feeling of being depleted. Many living with SIBO describe these layered symptoms as an ongoing struggle that feels increasingly burdensome if left untreated.

Proper intestinal movement, or motility, is a cornerstone in understanding and managing SIBO. The small intestine is designed to use rhythmic contractions, like waves, to move food along and prevent bacteria from staying too long. When this natural motility slows down–whether due to stress, nerve injuries, past surgeries, or conditions like hypothyroidism–bacteria have more time to settle and multiply excessively. This disruption often explains why SIBO tends to recur, even after successful treatment, if the root cause of slowed motility isn't properly addressed.

The role of bacterial toxins is another critical piece of the puzzle. These toxins, produced by the overgrowing bacteria, don't just escalate local inflammation–they also increase oxidative stress, ultimately weakening the intestinal lining. As a result, the body's natural ability to heal and maintain intestinal health is compromised. These factors make SIBO a particularly stubborn condition, with symptoms that can persist or worsen unless addressed through a thoughtful, multi-faceted approach.

Your immune system, too, has a vital role in maintaining balance within the gut. When it's weakened–whether by chronic illnesses, ongoing stress, or frequent use of medications like antibiotics–your body's ability to manage bacterial overgrowth diminishes. This sets in motion a vicious cycle: bacterial overgrowth harms intestinal health, further straining the immune system, and creating a self-perpetuating problem.

Diet plays a significant role, influencing intestinal health and the balance of gut bacteria. Diets low in fiber, high in processed foods, or lacking balance can tip the scales in favor of bacterial overgrowth. Even necessary treatments like antibiotics, which can work effectively to combat SIBO, sometimes disrupt the composition of gut bacteria. This disruption can leave your system vulnerable, creating ideal conditions for bacteria to flourish in the wrong part of the digestive system, triggering the cycle of SIBO once again.

Taking all of these factors into account highlights the importance of a comprehensive approach to managing SIBO: addressing motility issues, supporting immune health, improving the diet, and restoring balance to the gut bacteria, all while identifying and targeting individual causes to achieve lasting relief.

While SIBO primarily impacts the digestive system, its effects often ripple far beyond, influencing overall well-being. Many individuals–both men and women–notice a sharp drop in energy levels, shifts in mood, and a persistent sense of fatigue or unease that can disrupt daily life. It's completely understandable to feel frustrated or even disheartened by these challenges. Yet, it's crucial to know that SIBO is not an irreversible condition.

With the right tools and approach, you can regain control of your health and experience a renewed sense of vitality. The journey toward recovery often involves a thoughtful combination of dietary changes, probiotics, nutritional support, and targeted therapies. These are designed not just to alleviate symptoms but also to rebuild intestinal balance, fortify digestive health, and restore a stronger, healthier you.

This book has been carefully crafted to be your guide on this journey, offering clear, practical insights about SIBO and how to tackle it from several angles. Whether you're just beginning to explore solutions or have already traveled part of this path, within these pages you'll find the knowledge and support needed to understand your body, nurture your health, and enhance your quality of life. Wellness is not a distant goal–it's within your reach, and it starts with your commitment and care!

Symptoms of SIBO

Bacterial overgrowth in the small intestine (SIBO) can present a broad spectrum of symptoms that range in intensity from mild to severe. These symptoms can impact various systems in the body and may occur either chronically or intermittently. The following are the most common symptoms associated with this condition:

Gastrointestinal symptoms

‣ **Abdominal pain** is one of the primary symptoms of SIBO. It can vary in intensity and location and is often described as cramping or stabbing. The pain may worsen after eating or drinking and may be temporarily alleviated by a bowel movement.

‣ **Abdominal distention**: Another prevalent symptom of SIBO is abdominal distention, characterized by a bloated or swollen sensation in the abdomen that may be more noticeable after meals. Bloating can lead to discomfort and impact one's quality of life.

‣ **Flatulence**: Excessive gas production is a common symptom of SIBO. The abundance of bacteria in the small intestine generates gases like hydrogen and methane, leading to flatulence and frequent burping.

‣ **Diarrhea**: Chronic diarrhea is a frequent symptom of SIBO. It may manifest as loose, watery, or explosive stools and may be accompanied by fecal urgency and a sense of incomplete evacuation.

‣ **Constipation**: While less common than diarrhea, constipation can also manifest as a symptom. Bacterial overgrowth can disrupt intestinal motility, making it challenging to pass stool, which can result in constipation.

Symptoms related to nutrient absorption

‣ **Malabsorption of nutrients**: SIBO can impair the intestine's nutrient absorption capacity, leading to symptoms of malabsorption like fatty stools, postprandial bloating, nutritional deficiencies, weight loss, overall weakness, and deficiencies in vitamins and minerals.

‣ **Deficiencies in fat-soluble vitamins:** Malabsorption of fats due to SIBO can cause deficiencies in fat-soluble vitamins such as vitamins A, D, E, and K. This can impact bone health, immune function, and other metabolic processes.

‣ **Anemia:** SIBO can disrupt the absorption of iron and vitamin B12, potentially resulting in iron deficiency or pernicious anemia. Symptoms of anemia may include fatigue, weakness, pallor, and shortness of breath.

Symptoms related to the immune system

‣ **Inflammation:** SIBO can provoke an inflammatory response in the gut, characterized by abdominal pain, tenderness, and redness. Chronic inflammation can also contribute to systemic symptoms like fatigue and widespread bodily pain.

‣ **Food allergies and intolerances:** SIBO can harm the intestinal mucosa and increase intestinal permeability, allowing food allergens to enter the bloodstream. This can lead to food allergies and intolerances, resulting in symptoms such as rashes, itching, swelling, and breathing difficulties.

‣ **Autoimmune responses:** Some studies suggest that SIBO may trigger autoimmune reactions in specific individuals, potentially causing symptoms such as joint pain, chronic inflammation, fatigue, and other manifestations of auto-immune diseases.

Other symptoms

‣ **Fatigue:** SIBO can lead to chronic fatigue due to nutrient malabsorption and inflammation.

‣ **Skin problems:** Individuals with SIBO may encounter skin issues like rashes, redness, itching, ulcers, acne, rosacea, or eczema. These skin problems could stem from systemic inflammation and autoimmune responses associated with SIBO, necessitating medical assessment.

‣ **Headaches and migraines:** SIBO may trigger headaches and migraines in specific individuals, potentially due to inflammation and the release of inflammatory chemicals impacting the nervous system.

‣ **Sleep problems:** Many individuals with SIBO may struggle to sleep or maintain sleep. This could be attributed to abdominal discomfort, systemic inflammation, and neurotransmitter imbalances that can arise with SIBO.

‣ **Concentration and memory problems:** Some individuals with SIBO may encounter issues with concentration, difficulty retaining information, and brain fog. These challenges could be linked to chronic inflammation, malabsorption of essential nutrients for brain function, and neurotransmitter imbalances.

‣ **Neuropsychiatric symptoms:** In rare instances, SIBO may be correlated with neuropsychiatric symptoms like anxiety, depression, mood swings, cognitive challenges, or memory issues. These manifestations may arise from the excessive production of toxins by gut bacteria. If experiencing these symptoms, seeking medical attention is crucial for proper evaluation and treatment.

‣ **Musculoskeletal symptoms:** SIBO can induce pain, inflammation, or stiffness in joints, muscles, and soft tissues. These effects may stem from chronic inflammation, autoimmune responses, and neurotransmitter imbalances that can impact muscle and joint function.

‣ **Urinary symptoms:** Certain individuals with SIBO may display urinary symptoms such as increased urinary frequency, urgency, painful urination, or recurrent urinary tract infections. These symptoms could be attributed to inflammation and dysfunction in the autonomic nervous system.

‣ **Acid reflux:** SIBO can contribute to the development of acid reflux or gastroesophageal reflux disease (GERD). This can occur due to dysfunction of the lower esophageal sphincter (LES) caused by bacteria in the small intestine.

‣ **Respiratory symptoms**: Some individuals with SIBO may experience respiratory symptoms such as chronic cough, nasal congestion, recurrent sinusitis, or frequent respiratory infections. These symptoms may result from inflammation in the upper respiratory tract triggered by SIBO.

‣ **Neurological symptoms**: SIBO can impact the nervous system and lead to neurological symptoms like tingling or numbness in the limbs, dizziness, difficulty concentrating, or balance issues. These manifestations could be caused by inflammation, neurotransmitter imbalances, and the production of toxic substances by bacteria in the small intestine.

‣ **Thyroid problems**: SIBO has been linked to thyroid gland dysfunctions, such as hypothyroidism or hyperthyroidism. This association may be attributed to inflammation and hormonal imbalances that can arise with SIBO.

‣ **Menstrual problems**: In some women, SIBO can disrupt hormone balance and lead to menstrual issues like irregular periods, severe menstrual pain, or changes in menstrual flow. If experiencing these symptoms, seeking medical attention for proper evaluation and management is crucial.

It is essential to recognize that symptoms can vary among individuals, and not everyone with SIBO will encounter all the symptoms mentioned above. If you have concerns or suspect SIBO, I recommend seeking an evaluation by a medical professional for an accurate diagnosis.

Types of SIBO

Small Intestinal Bacterial Overgrowth (SIBO) is classified into distinct types based on the microorganisms involved and the underlying mechanisms contributing to its development. This classification offers a clearer understanding of the nature of SIBO and aids in identifying more targeted and effective treatment options.

‣ **SIBO with aerobic bacterial overgrowth:** In this type of SIBO, the predominant bacteria in the upper small intestine are aerobic, requiring oxygen to survive. These aerobic bacteria can infiltrate and proliferate, leading to symptoms such as bloating, gas, diarrhea, abdominal pain, and nutrient malabsorption. Common aerobic bacteria linked to this SIBO type include Escherichia coli, Klebsiella pneumoniae, and Enterococcus spp.

‣ **SIBO with anaerobic bacterial overgrowth:** In this type of SIBO, the primary bacteria in the large intestine, which have low oxygen levels, are anaerobic and can survive without oxygen. These anaerobic bacteria can migrate to the small intestine and multiply, causing symptoms akin to SIBO with aerobic bacteria. Common anaerobic bacteria associated with this type include Bacteroides spp., Clostridium spp., and Fusobacterium spp.

‣ **SIBO with mixed bacterial overgrowth:** This type of SIBO involves a combination of aerobic and anaerobic bacteria multiplying in the small intestine. Symptoms may overlap between the two kinds of bacteria. Treating this type of SIBO can be challenging as it necessitates a therapeutic approach targeting aerobic and anaerobic bacteria.

‣ **SIBO with methane-producing bacterial overgrowth:** In this type of SIBO, bacteria multiplying in the small intestine produce a significant amount of methane. Methane, a gas that can slow down intestinal motility, can lead to symptoms like constipation, bloating, and digestive discomfort. Common bacteria linked to this type of SIBO include Methanobrevibacter smithii and Methanosphaera stadtmanae. This SIBO variant is often associated with chronic constipation and may necessitate a specific treatment approach to lower methane levels.

‣ **SIBO associated with underlying diseases:** In certain instances, SIBO may be correlated with underlying conditions that impact the motility or functioning of the small intestine. These conditions include irritable bowel syndrome (IBS), inflammatory bowel disease (IBD), celiac disease, diabetes, and scleroderma. These ailments can influence intestinal motility and the functionality of the valves controlling bacterial flow from the large intestine to the small intestine, potentially predisposing individuals to SIBO development.

‣ **Post-surgical SIBO:** Certain abdominal surgeries, such as bariatric surgery, colectomy, or gastrectomy, can modify the anatomy and function of the small intestine, thereby increasing the likelihood of bacterial overgrowth. These surgeries can impact intestinal motility, decrease gastric acid production, or modify the function of intestinal valves, potentially allowing bacteria from the large intestine to migrate to the small intestine and proliferate extensively.

‣ **SIBO associated with inflammatory bowel disease (IBD):** Inflammatory bowel diseases, such as Crohn's disease and ulcerative colitis, may predispose individuals to SIBO. Chronic inflammation and alterations in intestinal motility can provide an environment for bacterial multiplication in the small intestine. Additionally, treatments utilized to manage IBD, like corticosteroids and immunosuppressants, can compromise the immune system and heighten the risk of SIBO.

‣ **SIBO is related to damage to the intestinal barrier:** The small intestine's lining is shielded by a protective layer that prevents bacteria from the large intestine from migrating into the small intestine. However, certain conditions and factors can compromise this barrier, such as excessive alcohol consumption, prolonged use of medications like non-steroidal anti-inflammatory drugs (NSAIDs) and antibiotics, untreated celiac disease, and intestinal infections. When the intestinal barrier is compromised, bacteria can infiltrate the small intestine, leading to SIBO.

‣ **SIBO related to motor dysfunction:** Intestinal motility involves the rhythmic contractions of intestinal muscles that facilitate the proper movement of food and bacteria through the digestive tract. If intestinal motility is dysfunctional, food may stagnate, and the small intestine may empty slowly, creating an environment conducive to bacterial overgrowth.

Conditions that can impact intestinal motility include irritable bowel syndrome (IBS), Parkinson's disease, scleroderma, and dysfunction of the vagus nerve.

‣ **SIBO related to hypochlorhydria or reduced stomach acid levels**: Stomach acid plays a crucial role in digestion and eliminating harmful bacteria. When stomach acid levels are low, bacteria can survive the journey through the stomach and reach the small intestine, where they can proliferate and lead to SIBO. Conditions that can result in reduced stomach acid levels include atrophic gastritis, prolonged use of proton pump inhibitor (PPI) medications, and Helicobacter pylori infection.

‣ **Coeliac disease-related SIBO**: Coeliac disease is an auto-immune condition triggered by the consumption of gluten, which provokes an inflammatory response in the small intestine. This chronic inflammation can disrupt intestinal motility and compromise the protective barrier of the intestine, facilitating bacterial overgrowth. Individuals with untreated or uncontrolled coeliac disease are at an elevated risk of developing SIBO.

‣ **SIBO related to pancreatic insufficiency**: The pancreas produces digestive enzymes crucial for breaking down food in the small intestine. When pancreatic insufficiency occurs, insufficient enzymes are produced, impacting proper food digestion and creating an environment for bacterial proliferation in the small intestine. Pancreatic insufficiency can be triggered by conditions like chronic pancreatitis, cystic fibrosis, or surgical removal of the pancreas.

‣ **SIBO related to yeast overgrowth**: While SIBO is primarily linked to bacterial overgrowth, yeasts like Candida albicans can also overgrow in the small intestine. These yeasts can proliferate and induce symptoms akin to SIBO, like bloating, gas, and digestive discomfort. Treatment for yeast-related SIBO typically involves antifungal therapy and dietary modifications to curb yeast growth.

‣ **SIBO is related to gut dysbiosis**: Gut dysbiosis refers to an imbalance in the composition of the gut microbiota, encompassing the bacteria and other microorganisms inhabiting the gut. When dysbiosis occurs, it can lead to an overgrowth of specific bacteria in the small intestine, fostering the development of SIBO. Factors contributing to gut dysbiosis include prolonged antibiotic use, an unhealthy diet, chronic stress, and other diseases or conditions disrupting the microbiota balance.

‣ **Achalasia-related SIBO**: Achalasia is an esophageal disorder characterized by impaired muscle function that hinders food passage into the stomach. This dysfunction can result in food and acid reflux into the esophagus, affecting intestinal motility and increasing susceptibility to SIBO development. Achalasia can also lead to food stagnation in the esophagus, creating an environment conducive to bacterial growth.

‣ **SIBO related to intestinal hypomotility**: Intestinal hypomotility refers to a reduction in muscle movements within the intestine, leading to the stagnation of food and bacteria in the small intestine. This creates an environment conducive to bacterial overgrowth and the onset of SIBO. Intestinal hypomotility may be linked to various conditions, such as hypothyroidism, Parkinson's disease, multiple sclerosis, and other neurological disorders.

‣ **SIBO related to excessive laxative use**: Prolonged use of laxatives can impact intestinal motility and disrupt the gut microbiota, increasing the likelihood of developing SIBO. Laxatives can induce dependency and diminish the gut's natural ability to propel food and bacteria through the digestive tract effectively. This can facilitate bacterial proliferation in the small intestine and trigger SIBO symptoms.

‣ **SIBO related to gastrointestinal surgery**: Certain surgical procedures in the gastrointestinal tract can modify the normal anatomy or function of the intestine, potentially leading to SIBO development. For instance, gastric bypass or bowel resection surgery may influence intestinal motility or nutrient absorption capacity, creating favorable conditions for bacterial overgrowth in the small intestine.

▸ **SIBO related to short bowel syndrome:** Short bowel syndrome is a condition where a significant portion of the small intestine has been surgically removed due to disease, trauma, or congenital malformation. With a reduced length of the small intestine, there may be diminished nutrient absorption capacity and impaired intestinal motility, potentially fostering the development of SIBO.

▸ **Diabetes-related SIBO:** The prevalence of SIBO has been higher in individuals with type 1 and type 2 diabetes. Diabetes can impact gut motility and the function of the nervous system, which regulates bowel movements. Furthermore, elevated blood glucose levels can create a conducive environment for bacterial growth in the small intestine.

▸ **SIBO related to excessive consumption of fermentable carbohydrates:** Certain carbohydrates, such as FODMAPs (fermentable oligosaccharides, disaccharides, monosaccharides, and polyols), are fermented by gut bacteria. In susceptible people, overconsumption of these fermentable carbohydrates can lead to SIBO symptoms, as bacteria metabolize them and produce gas and other fermentation byproducts that may cause digestive discomfort.

▸ **Immunodeficiency-related SIBO:** Conditions affecting the immune system, such as HIV/AIDS or immunoglobulin deficiency, can compromise the gut's immune function and predispose individuals to SIBO development. A weakened immune system may struggle to control bacterial overgrowth in the small intestine.

Causes of SIBO

Bacterial overgrowth in the small intestine can result from a variety of causes, often stemming from a combination of contributing factors.

▸ **Impaired intestinal motility:** The small intestine undergoes rhythmic movements known as peristalsis, aiding in the transportation of food and bacteria into the colon. Dysfunctions in intestinal motility, such as those seen in Parkinson's disease, irritable bowel syndrome (IBS), or scleroderma, can result in bacterial accumulation in the small intestine.

‣ **Abnormal anatomy of the gastrointestinal tract**: Certain medical conditions, such as abdominal adhesions, intestinal obstructions, or fistulas, can modify the normal anatomy of the gastrointestinal tract, leading to bacterial stagnation in the small intestine.

‣ **Ileocaecal sphincter dysfunction**: The ileocaecal sphincter serves as a valve between the small intestine and the colon, primarily preventing colonic bacteria from refluxing into the small intestine. If this sphincter malfunctions, bacterial reflux into the small intestine can contribute to SIBO.

‣ **Enzyme deficits**: Inadequate production of pancreatic and biliary enzymes can impact the proper digestion of food in the small intestine, accumulating undigested nutrients that serve as a substrate for bacterial growth.

‣ **Immune system dysfunction**: A compromised immune system, whether resulting from autoimmune conditions, immune deficiencies, or immunosuppressive drugs, can facilitate bacterial proliferation in the small intestine.

‣ **Prolonged use of medications**: Certain medications, like proton pump inhibitors (PPIs), broad-spectrum antibiotics, and opioids, can disrupt the bacterial balance in the gut and promote bacterial overgrowth.

‣ **Previous abdominal surgery**: Abdominal surgeries, such as bowel resection or bariatric surgery, can modify the structure and function of the small intestine, heightening the risk of SIBO.

‣ **Hypochlorhydria**: This is a condition characterized by

insufficient hydrochloric acid production in the stomach. Hydrochloric acid plays a crucial role in sterilizing bacteria entering the small intestine from the stomach. In cases of hypochlorhydria, bacteria can survive and multiply in the small intestine, contributing to SIBO.

‣ **Excessive consumption of fermentable carbohydrates**: Fermentable carbohydrates, such as those found in certain foods, such as fructose, lactose, and sorbitol, can ferment in the gut, providing a substrate for bacterial growth. Over-consumption of these carbohydrates may contribute to the development of SIBO in susceptible individuals.

‣ **Dysfunction of the enteric nervous system**: Often referred to as the "second brain," the enteric nervous system oversees numerous digestive functions. If it malfunctions, such as Parkinson's disease or autonomic neuropathy, it can disrupt motility and bacterial balance in the small intestine, predisposing individuals to SIBO.

‣ **Dietary and lifestyle factors**: Certain dietary choices may contribute to SIBO development. For instance, a low-fiber diet can impact intestinal motility and foster bacterial growth. Chronic stress can also disrupt normal digestive system function and heighten the risk of SIBO.

‣ **Underlying diseases**: Specific underlying conditions can make individuals more susceptible to SIBO. These conditions include inflammatory bowel disease (IBD), celiac disease, type 1 diabetes, and Crohn's disease. Such diseases can alter bowel function and create an environment favorable for bacterial growth in the small intestine.

‣ **Lymphatic system dysfunction**: The lymphatic system is vital in eliminating bacteria and waste from the intestine. If it is dysfunctional, such as after surgery or due to lymphatic obstruction, bacterial accumulation may occur in the small intestine.

‣ **Congenital anatomical alterations**: Some individuals may have congenital malformations of the gastrointestinal tract that predispose them to SIBO. These malformations may involve an abnormally short length of the small intestine or an atypical configuration of the intestinal loops.

‣ **Dysfunction of digestive secretions**: Gastric juices and pancreatic enzymes are essential for proper food digestion and absorption. Reduced production or release of these secretions can disrupt the bacterial balance in the small intestine, potentially contributing to SIBO development.

‣ **Excessive alcohol consumption**: Chronic and excessive alcohol consumption can harm the intestinal mucosa and impact gastrointestinal motility. This can increase the likelihood of SIBO by promoting bacterial overgrowth in the small intestine.

‣ **Abdominal radiotherapy**: Radiotherapy directed at the abdominal region as part of cancer treatment can damage the intestinal mucosa and disrupt the normal bacterial flora. This disruption can create an environment favorable for SIBO development.

‣ **Hormonal changes**: Certain hormonal fluctuations can impact intestinal motility and bacterial balance in the small intestine, raising the risk of SIBO. For instance, an increased incidence of SIBO has been noted in pregnant women due to fluctuating hormone levels.

‣ **Chronic stress**: Prolonged stress can detrimentally affect digestive health. Chronic stress can modify intestinal motility and immune function, potentially contributing to SIBO development.

‣ **Excessive antibiotic use**: Extended or excessive antibiotic use can disrupt the natural gut bacterial flora, permitting the proliferation of unwanted bacteria in the small intestine.

‣ **Use of proton pump inhibitors (PPIs)**: PPIs, such as Omeprazole, Nexium, Prevacid, Protonix, and Aciphex, are commonly prescribed to reduce stomach acid production and treat conditions like acid reflux and ulcers. Nonetheless, prolonged use of PPIs may disturb the small intestine's bacterial balance, heightening the risk of SIBO.

▸ **Neuromuscular diseases**: Certain neuromuscular conditions, such as amyotrophic lateral sclerosis (ALS) and Parkinson's disease, can impact gut motor function and potentially predispose individuals to SIBO.

Possible Long-Term Complications

This section is designed to offer clear guidance and effectively highlight potential risks, with an emphasis on prevention. By doing so, you can take proactive steps to safeguard your well-being and minimize the likelihood of complications.

If SIBO is not properly treated, it can result in a range of complications and adverse effects on the body, detailed as follows:

▸ **Malabsorption of nutrients**: SIBO can disrupt the proper absorption of nutrients in the small intestine. Excessive bacteria can harm intestinal cells and hinder the production of digestive enzymes necessary for food breakdown and nutrient absorption. This can result in nutritional deficiencies, weight loss, fatigue, anemia, and other symptoms associated with malabsorption.

▸ **Irritable Bowel Syndrome (IBS)**: SIBO has been linked to an increased likelihood of developing IBS. The surplus bacteria can trigger inflammation and irritation in the small intestine lining, causing symptoms like abdominal pain, bloating, alterations in bowel habits, and general discomfort.

▸ **Malnutrition**: SIBO can impede the absorption of fats and fat-soluble vitamins, such as vitamins A, D, E, and K. This can lead to deficiencies in these vitamins and subsequent malabsorption of fats, resulting in fatty stools, vitamin deficiencies, and weight loss.

▸ **Food intolerances**: Excessive bacteria in the small intestine can trigger adverse reactions to specific foods, potentially resulting in the development of food intolerances like lactose intolerance, gluten intolerance, or other food sensitivities.

▶ **Recurrent bacterial overgrowth syndrome:** In certain instances, SIBO can evolve into a chronic, recurrent condition. This means that, despite treatment, bacteria may repeatedly overgrow in the small intestine, leading to the recurrence of symptoms.

▶ **Compromised immune system:** Chronic SIBO can impact immune system function. Excess bacteria can continuously stimulate an immune response, potentially causing chronic inflammation and elevating the risk of autoimmune diseases or inflammatory disorders.

▶ **Persistent gastrointestinal symptoms:** SIBO can trigger chronic and enduring gastrointestinal symptoms, such as diarrhea, constipation, bloating, flatulence, and general malaise. These symptoms can significantly impact an individual's quality of life and impede their ability to carry out daily activities.

▶ **Damage to the intestinal barrier:** SIBO can harm the intestinal barrier, the protective layer of cells lining the intestine. This damage can permit bacteria and toxins to breach the barrier and enter the bloodstream, leading to increased intestinal permeability or "leaky gut." Such permeability can incite inflammatory responses in the body and contribute to developing autoimmune diseases and other inflammatory disorders.

▶ **Extraintestinal symptoms:** SIBO impacts the gastro-intestinal tract and can manifest symptoms beyond the digestive system. Individuals with SIBO have reported experiencing symptoms like chronic fatigue, muscle and joint pain, headaches, memory and concentration issues, irritability, and depression. These symptoms may stem from systemic inflammation and toxins produced by excess bacteria.

‣ **Increased inflammation:** Chronic SIBO can foster a state of persistent inflammation in the body. Excessive bacteria can release toxins and trigger an inflammatory reaction, potentially harming various body systems and organs. Chronic inflammation has been linked to an elevated risk of cardiovascular disease, autoimmune disorders, and other health complications.

‣ **Complications associated with other medical conditions:** SIBO can exacerbate symptoms and complications of different medical conditions, such as inflammatory bowel disease (IBD), leaky gut syndrome, celiac disease, and diabetes. Excessive bacteria can amplify inflammation and digestive issues in these pre-existing conditions.

‣ **Gut microbiota imbalance:** SIBO can disturb the balance of the gut microbiota, the community of beneficial microorganisms residing in the gastrointestinal tract. Bacterial overgrowth can adversely impact the diversity and composition of the microbiota, influencing digestive health, the immune system, and overall well-being.

‣ **Recurrence of urinary tract infections:** Bacteria that overgrow in the small intestine can migrate into the urinary tract, heightening the risk of recurrent infections. This is because bacteria can potentially colonize the urethra and bladder, leading to repeated infections.

‣ **Hormonal dysregulation:** Chronic SIBO can disrupt the body's production and balance of hormones. Excessive bacteria can influence hormone metabolism and endocrine gland function, resulting in hormonal imbalances. These imbalances may manifest as symptoms such as changes in the menstrual cycle, decreased libido, fertility issues, and dysregulation of other hormonal systems.

‣ **Increased risk of metabolic diseases:** SIBO has been linked to a higher risk of developing metabolic diseases, such as insulin resistance, type 2 diabetes, and obesity. Bacterial overgrowth may disrupt blood sugar regulation and lipid metabolism, potentially predisposing individuals to these metabolic conditions.

‣ **Nervous system-related complications:** Some people with SIBO may experience nervous system-related complications like peripheral neuropathy, migraines, and mood disorders. SIBO can impact the gut-brain axis, affecting neurological function and mood.

‣ **Vitamin and mineral deficiencies:** SIBO can impede the proper absorption of essential vitamins and minerals crucial for optimal bodily function. This interference can lead to nutrient deficiencies such as vitamin B12, iron, magnesium, and zinc, negatively impacting overall health and well-being.

‣ **Impact on mental health:** Chronic SIBO can significantly influence mental health and emotional well-being. Persistent digestive symptoms, physical discomfort, and SIBO-related complications can contribute to stress, anxiety, and depression. Furthermore, the gut-brain connection and imbalance in the gut microbiota can affect the production of mood-related neurotransmitters.

‣ **Food allergies:** SIBO may contribute to the development of food allergies. Bacterial overgrowth can harm the intestinal mucosa and trigger an inflammatory response, making the immune system hypersensitive to certain foods. This can result in the onset of food allergies or the exacerbation of existing intolerances.

‣ **Skin problems:** Individuals with SIBO may experience skin issues like acne, rosacea, eczema, and psoriasis. This is believed to be linked to the gut-skin axis, the connection between the gut and the skin. Imbalances in the gut microbiota and inflammation due to SIBO can impact skin health and contribute to skin problems.

‣ **Liver problems:** SIBO can influence liver function and contribute to liver diseases such as non-alcoholic hepatic steatosis (fatty liver) and hepatitis. The presence of excessive bacteria in the small intestine can elevate the burden of toxins and metabolic by-products that the liver must process, potentially impairing liver function.

‣ **Gallbladder problems**: SIBO can impact gallbladder function and contribute to gallstone formation. Excessive bacteria can disrupt bile composition and promote gallstone development. Furthermore, chronic SIBO may be linked to a higher occurrence of cholecystitis, a gallbladder inflammation.

‣ **Kidney complications**: Chronic SIBO may be linked to an elevated risk of developing kidney disease, such as chronic kidney disease. It is believed that the presence of excessive bacteria in the small intestine may increase the load of toxins and metabolic products that the kidneys must filter, potentially straining their function and contributing to the onset of kidney disease.

‣ **Impact on bone health**: Some studies have indicated a potential correlation between chronic SIBO and compromised bone health. It is theorized that bacterial imbalance in the gut could disrupt calcium absorption and metabolism, adversely affecting bone density and heightening the risk of osteoporosis and bone fractures.

Reduction of Symptoms and Prevention

SIBO is a condition marked by an abnormal overgrowth of bacteria in the small intestine, which can cause a range of uncomfortable symptoms and negatively affect overall well-being. Fortunately, there are effective strategies available to both alleviate these symptoms and prevent their recurrence. These include:

‣ **Low fermentable carbohydrate diet**: SIBO is linked to the fermentation of carbohydrates in the small intestine, resulting in gas and related symptoms. A diet low in fermentable carbohydrates, like a low-FODMAP diet (Fermentable Oligosaccharides, Disaccharides, Mono-saccharides, and Polyols), helps alleviate these symptoms by constraining the food source for bacteria. These fermentable carbohydrates are challenging to digest and can fuel bacterial proliferation in the small intestine.

‣ **Probiotics**: Probiotics are beneficial bacteria that help rebalance the gut flora. However, when treating SIBO, caution must be exercised when selecting probiotics, as certain types may exacerbate symptoms in some individuals.

‣ **Adequate nutrition**: Maintaining a balanced and consistent diet is crucial for fostering optimal gut health. This entails consuming a diverse array of nourishing foods rich in fiber and antioxidants while minimizing the intake of processed foods and those high in saturated fats.

‣ **Stress management**: Prolonged stress can negatively impact gut health and exacerbate SIBO symptoms. Engaging in stress management practices such as meditation, yoga, tai chi, or cognitive behavioral therapy can alleviate symptoms and avert recurrence.

‣ **Treatment of underlying diseases**: SIBO may be linked to other underlying diseases or conditions that impact the digestive system's functionality, such as inflammatory bowel disease, celiac disease, or lower esophageal sphincter dysfunction. Managing and treating these conditions can aid in symptom reduction and SIBO prevention.

‣ **Intestinal motility**: Intestinal motility refers to the synchronized movement of muscles in the digestive tract that facilitates food passage through the system. Delayed intestinal motility can contribute to SIBO development. In certain instances, supplements or prokinetic drugs may enhance intestinal motility and prevent excessive bacterial accumulation in the small intestine.

‣ **Avoid excessive alcohol consumption and smoking**: Excessive alcohol intake and smoking have adverse effects on gut health and heighten the risk of SIBO development. Limiting or eliminating alcohol consumption and refraining from smoking is advantageous for SIBO prevention and treatment.

‣ **Treatment of digestive dysfunctions**: Some individuals may experience digestive dysfunctions that contribute to the onset of SIBO, such as pancreatic insufficiency or low stomach acidity. These conditions impede proper food digestion and can foster bacterial growth in the small intestine. Addressing these dysfunctions with enzyme supplements or hydrochloric acid aids in symptom alleviation.

‣ **Avoid excessive use of medications that affect gut flora**: Certain medications, such as broad-spectrum antibiotics, proton pump inhibitors (PPIs), and antacids, can disrupt gut flora balance and increase SIBO risk. It is crucial to use these medications only when necessary, under a doctor's prescription and supervision. Consider natural alternatives or therapies that minimize the impact on gut flora whenever possible.

‣ **Nutritional supplements**: Some nutritional supplements, like oregano oil, can be beneficial in treating and preventing SIBO.

‣ **Proper food hygiene**: Ensuring food safety is essential in preventing bacterial infections that may contribute to SIBO development. To prevent cross-contamination, thoroughly wash fruits and vegetables before consumption, handle and store food correctly, and opt for fresh, high-quality food.

‣ **Identifying and treating food intolerances**: Individuals with SIBO may have food intolerances, such as lactose or gluten intolerance, that can trigger digestive symptoms. Identifying and eliminating trigger foods can help alleviate symptoms and provide relief.

‣ **Follow a holistic approach to gut health**: Gut health is a multifaceted and intricate system. In addition to the above aspects, maintaining an overall healthy lifestyle is essential. Effective SIBO treatment involves a holistic approach encompassing dietary changes, supplements, herbal remedies, prescribed medications under medical supervision, adequate sleep, hydration, regular exercise, and stress management. These practices positively impact gut health, aiding in SIBO and recurrence prevention.

‣ **Maintain a proper balance of gut bacteria**: Besides addressing excess bacteria in the small intestine, it is crucial to promote a healthy balance of gut bacteria overall. Consuming foods rich in natural probiotics, such as plain yogurt, kefir, sauerkraut, or kimchi, helps foster a healthy gut environment. Additionally, foods high in prebiotic fiber, like green leafy vegetables, asparagus, and artichokes, provide nutrients that nourish the beneficial bacteria in the gut.

‣ **Avoid excessive consumption of processed foods and refined sugars**. Processed foods containing refined sugars and sweeteners encourage bacterial growth in the small intestine. A diet centered on whole, fresh foods that are nutrient-dense and low in added sugars and sweeteners can help reduce SIBO symptoms and promote optimal gut health.

‣ **Regular medical follow-up**: Regular professional follow-up is essential to evaluate the effectiveness of treatment and make necessary adjustments. Doctors may conduct follow-up tests, such as breath tests or duodenal aspirate cultures, to determine treatment success and whether SIBO has been resolved.

‣ **Education and understanding**: It can be beneficial to understand the factors contributing to SIBO development, associated symptoms, and prevention strategies.

Additional Guidelines

It is crucial to avoid self-medication and always seek guidance from a healthcare professional before taking any medication. Your doctor, pharmacist, or healthcare specialist is the most qualified person to evaluate your individual case and recommend the most appropriate treatment for your specific needs.

Diagnostic Medical Tests

Medical diagnostic tests are vital for confirming the diagnosis. Below are some of the key tests commonly used to detect SIBO:

‣ **Lactulose breath test**: This is one of the most commonly used methods to diagnose SIBO. The person swallows a solution of lactulose, a non-digestible sugar, and breath samples are taken at regular intervals over several hours. Lactulose is fermented by bacteria in the small intestine, producing gases like hydrogen and methane, which can be detected in the breath. A significant increase in these gases indicates a potential bacterial overgrowth in the small intestine.

‣ **Glucose breath test**: Similar to the lactulose breath test, this test involves ingesting a glucose solution instead of lactulose. Glucose is also fermented by bacteria in the small intestine, leading to the production of gases detectable in the breath. This test can be an alternative to the lactulose breath test.

‣ **Duodenal aspirate culture**: In this test, an endoscopy is performed to collect a sample of fluid or contents from the small intestine. The sample is then sent to a laboratory for culture and analysis to detect bacterial growth. However, this method may have limitations, as bacteria may not grow properly in the culture medium, or there may be discrepancies in the interpretation of the results.

‣ **Duodenal aspirate test with bacteria count**: This test also involves an endoscopy to obtain a sample from the small intestine. The sample is analyzed in the laboratory to determine the quantity of bacteria present. A high bacterial count in the small intestine may suggest bacterial overgrowth.

‣ **Duodenal aspirate test with Gram stain**: This test is conducted similarly to the duodenal aspirate test mentioned earlier, but instead of counting the bacteria, a Gram stain is applied to the sample. The Gram stain enables visualization of the bacteria in the sample and identification of their composition and characteristics. This can offer additional insights into the bacteria present in the small intestine.

‣ **Duodenal aspirate culture and biopsy test**: This test involves obtaining an aspirate and biopsy sample from the small intestine during endoscopy. The samples are then sent to a laboratory for culture and analyzed for bacterial growth and composition. This can provide more comprehensive information about the bacteria in the small intestine.

‣ **PCR (polymerase chain reaction) test**: This molecular test detects bacterial DNA in a small intestine sample. It can identify and quantify specific bacterial strains, offering more precise information about the types of bacteria present in the small intestine.

‣ **D-xylose absorption test**: This test assesses the small intestine's ability to absorb D-xylose, a sugar typically absorbed in the small intestine. A dose of D-xylose is administered, and the absorption level is measured in the blood or urine. An abnormally low result may indicate minor intestinal dysfunction, potentially due to bacterial over-growth.

‣ **Bowel transit test**: This test evaluates the speed at which food moves through the digestive system. A capsule containing radiopaque tracers is ingested, and X-rays are taken periodically to monitor the tracers' progress through the intestines. An unusually rapid bowel transit rate may suggest potential SIBO.

‣ **Stool protein electrophoresis test**: This test measures protein levels in stool to identify inflammation in the intestine. Inflammation could indicate an imbalance of bacteria in the small intestine.

‣ **Intestinal permeability test**: This test gauges the intestine's ability to maintain an effective intestinal barrier. A solution of lactulose and mannitol is orally administered, and the levels of these sugars in the urine are monitored over a specific timeframe. An elevated lactulose level in the urine may signify increased intestinal permeability, which could be linked to SIBO.

It is important to emphasize that each diagnostic test for SIBO has its own specific advantages and limitations. The choice of the most appropriate test will depend on various factors, including its availability, the expertise of the physician, and the individual's unique characteristics, such as their medical history and specific symptoms.

In addition, it is crucial that these tests are conducted under the supervision of a physician specializing in digestive disorders. This approach ensures an accurate interpretation of the results and the development of an optimal, personalized treatment plan tailored to each case.

Warning Signs

SIBO can present with a wide range of symptoms, but certain ones are considered warning signs. These symptoms may suggest complications or more serious conditions related to the disease, making prompt medical evaluation critically important.

‣ **Rectal bleeding**: Rectal bleeding or blood in the stool may signal inflammation, damage to the bowel lining, or potentially a severe complication like an ulcer or bowel perforation. This could be a result of SIBO and requires medical evaluation.

‣ **Unexplained weight loss**: Unexplained weight loss could be a red flag and may indicate nutrient malabsorption due to SIBO. If you are experiencing significant weight loss without a clear cause, it is crucial to seek medical attention to investigate other potential underlying issues, such as cancer.

‣ **Anemia**: SIBO can disrupt the absorption of iron and other essential vitamins and minerals, leading to anemia. Symptoms of anemia may include fatigue, weakness, pallor, and shortness of breath. If you are experiencing these symptoms, seeking medical attention to assess your iron levels and receive appropriate treatment is essential.

‣ **Severe or persistent abdominal pain:** While SIBO can lead to abdominal pain, experiencing severe or persistent abdominal pain, particularly when accompanied by other symptoms like fever, vomiting, or severe bloating, warrants immediate medical attention. These symptoms could indicate a serious complication such as bowel obstruction, perforation, appendicitis, or a severe bacterial infection.

‣ **Changes in bowel habits:** Significant alterations in bowel habits, such as severe diarrhea or persistent constipation, should prompt medical attention. These changes may suggest impaired bowel function due to SIBO or other conditions requiring treatment.

‣ **Neurological symptoms:** In rare instances, SIBO can trigger neurological symptoms like numbness, tingling, muscle weakness, difficulty walking, or coordination issues. These symptoms may indicate a complication known as small intestinal bacterial overgrowth with D-lactate overproduction (SIBOS-D). If you experience these symptoms, immediate medical attention is advised.

‣ **Persistent high fever:** A persistent high fever, particularly when accompanied by symptoms like severe abdominal pain or bloating, necessitates immediate medical attention. Fever could signal a severe intestinal infection, such as perforation or a generalized infection.

‣ **Persistent vomiting:** Continuous vomiting can serve as a red flag and may indicate a bowel obstruction or a severe complication of SIBO. If you are experiencing persistent vomiting, especially when accompanied by severe abdominal pain or the inability to retain fluids, immediate medical attention is recommended.

‣ **Severe dehydration:** Prolonged diarrhea resulting from SIBO can lead to dehydration. Symptoms of dehydration include dry mouth, intense thirst, dizziness, extreme fatigue, and reduced urine output. If you are experiencing these symptoms, seeking medical attention to receive adequate hydration is crucial.

‣ **Severe respiratory symptoms**: In certain instances, SIBO may be linked to severe respiratory issues, such as aspiration pneumonia. If you experience shortness of breath, chest pain, or difficulty breathing, immediate medical attention is advised.

‣ **Pain in the right shoulder**: Pain in the right shoulder could be a symptom of a severe complication of SIBO, such as a liver abscess. If you are experiencing intense pain in your right shoulder, prompt medical attention is necessary.

‣ **Chest pain**: SIBO can trigger inflammation in the intestine and diaphragm, leading to chest pain. If you encounter sudden, severe, or persistent chest pain, immediate medical attention is crucial, as it could signify a severe complication.

‣ **Gallbladder problems**: SIBO can impact gallbladder function, resulting in symptoms like right-sided abdominal pain, nausea, vomiting, and digestive issues related to fat digestion. If you experience these symptoms, it is essential to seek medical attention to thoroughly evaluate gallbladder function.

‣ **Low back pain**: SIBO can cause inflammation in the intestines, affecting the nerves in the lower back and causing chronic or recurring low back pain. If you are experiencing persistent or severe low back pain, seeking medical attention for a proper evaluation is essential.

‣ **Extreme fatigue**: Severe and enduring fatigue can be a concerning symptom associated with SIBO. If you experience debilitating fatigue that does not improve with rest, seeking medical attention for a thorough evaluation and management is essential.

If you develop any of these symptoms, it is essential to promptly consult a medical professional for a thorough evaluation.

FREQUENTLY ASKED QUESTIONS

Navigating the intricate world of health can feel overwhelming, especially when faced with a diagnosis that affects both physical and emotional well-being. In such moments, many questions naturally arise: What does this mean for me? What options are available? How will my daily life change? Uncertainty and concern are common. Here, you'll discover practical and direct insights to help you make confident, informed choices.

This chapter was created to offer support and provide clear, straightforward tools to guide you through this journey. In today's era of abundant information, distinguishing reliable knowledge from content that might cause confusion is vital. With this in mind, I've compiled evidence-based guidance to help you navigate uncertainty with greater clarity.

The format of this resource prioritizes accessibility, addressing common concerns faced by individuals and families alike. Each explanation is concise, clear, and aimed at empowering you to make decisions that align with your overall well-being.

While the material here is designed to assist, it is not a substitute for personalized advice from healthcare professionals. Consulting your doctor for guidance tailored to your specific needs remains essential, especially to address challenges unique to your situation.

Through these pages, my goal is to foster calm, confidence, and reassurance so that you can approach your circumstances with strength and resolve. I hope this resource inspires you and provides the valuable tools necessary to manage your health effectively and confidently.

135 FAQs about SIBO

1. What is SIBO?

SIBO refers to bacterial overgrowth in the small intestine. It is a condition with excess bacteria in the small intestine, which causes digestive and nutrient absorption problems, among others.

2. What are the common symptoms of SIBO?

Symptoms may include bloating, abdominal pain, diarrhea, constipation, gas, nausea, and fatigue. Malabsorption of nutrients can also lead to nutritional deficiencies.

3. What causes SIBO?

Causes can vary but often include intestinal motility problems, changes in the intestine's pH, alterations in the immune system, or previous minor bowel surgery. It may also be associated with conditions such as irritable bowel syndrome (IBS), celiac disease, or diabetes.

4. How is SIBO diagnosed?

There are several medical tests to diagnose SIBO. The lactulose or glucose breath test measures the hydrogen or methane exhaled after carbohydrate ingestion. A significant increase indicates the presence of bacteria in the small intestine.

5. What is the treatment for SIBO?

Standard treatment includes antibiotics, such as rifaximin, to reduce the amount of bacteria. Dietary changes, probiotics, and nutritional supplements are also recommended to address deficiencies.

6. What role does diet play in the management of SIBO?

Diet is crucial in the management of SIBO. Low FODMAP or SIBO-specific diets help reduce symptoms by limiting foods that fuel bacterial overgrowth.

7. Can SIBO be cured?

While symptoms can be remitted, SIBO can recur, primarily if the underlying causes are not adequately addressed. A comprehensive approach that includes treatment, dietary adjustments, and management of underlying conditions helps prevent relapses.

8. What complications can SIBO cause if left untreated?
If left untreated, SIBO can lead to malabsorption of nutrients, which can cause malnutrition, unintended weight loss, and vitamin and mineral deficiencies, among others.

9. How does SIBO affect the quality of life?
The symptoms of SIBO can be debilitating and significantly affect a person's quality of life, interfering with daily activities and general well-being.

10. Is the use of probiotics recommended?
The use of probiotics in SIBO is a debated topic. Some people may benefit from certain types of probiotics; in other cases, they may worsen symptoms. It is essential to consult with a healthcare professional to determine the best approach.

11. What is the difference between hydrogen and methane SIBO?
SIBO can be classified according to the gas that the excess bacteria produce: hydrogen or methane. Hydrogen SIBO is usually associated with diarrhea, while methane SIBO is more often associated with constipation. Breath tests measure these gases to help determine the type of SIBO present.

12. Can stress influence the development or worsening of SIBO?
Yes, stress affects intestinal motility and immune system function, which may contribute to the development or worsening of SIBO. Stress management techniques can be part of a comprehensive approach to treatment.

13. Are there risk factors for developing SIBO?
Some risk factors include diseases that affect intestinal motility, such as scleroderma, long-term use of proton pump inhibitors, previous intestinal surgery, and conditions that cause intestinal obstruction.

14. Does SIBO affect children and adults equally?
Although SIBO can affect people of all ages, it is more common

in adults. In children, it may be related to congenital conditions or chronic diseases.

15. How does SIBO affect the absorption of fats and vitamins?

SIBO can interfere with normal digestion and absorption of fats, leading to steatorrhea (fatty stools). Fat malabsorption can also cause deficiencies in fat-soluble vitamins (A, D, E, and K).

16. Is SIBO related to irritable bowel syndrome (IBS)?

Many people with IBS also have SIBO, and the symptoms may overlap. Some studies suggest that SIBO may be an underlying cause of IBS symptoms in certain people. Treating SIBO can significantly relieve IBS symptoms.

17. What role do antibiotics play in the treatment of SIBO?

Antibiotics, especially those that act locally in the intestine, such as rifaximin, reduce the number of bacteria in the small intestine. Following the regimen prescribed by a physician is essential to minimize the risk of antibiotic resistance.

18. What role does the FODMAP diet play?

A low FODMAP diet helps reduce symptoms by limiting certain fermentable carbohydrates that bacteria in the small intestine can use as food.

19. Are there natural or complementary treatments?

Many seek complementary treatments, such as antimicrobial herbs (e.g., oregano oil, garlic) or digestive supplements.

20. Can SIBO be a recurrent problem?

Yes, SIBO can recur, mainly if the underlying causes are not addressed. Regular follow-up with a healthcare professional and a comprehensive treatment approach help to manage recurrence.

21. How does SIBO influence the immune system?

SIBO can weaken the immune system by compromising the intestinal barrier, allowing bacteria and their products to enter the bloodstream, and altering the microbial balance, increasing susceptibility to infection.

22. How does SIBO affect mental health?

There is a strong connection between the gut and the brain, known as the gut-brain axis. SIBO can contribute to symptoms of anxiety and depression due to the production of bacterial toxins and malabsorption of nutrients essential for brain health.

23. What role does intestinal motility play in the development of SIBO?

Adequate intestinal motility is crucial for cleansing the small intestine of bacteria and waste. Dysfunction in motility, such as gastroparesis or irritable bowel syndrome, may contribute to the development of SIBO.

24. Can SIBO cause food intolerances?

Yes, SIBO can lead to food intolerances due to intestinal inflammation and mucosal disruption, which could lead to an immune response against certain foods.

25. How is SIBO related to celiac disease?

Celiac disease can damage the small intestine's lining, affecting intestinal motility and bacterial balance. This can predispose to the development of SIBO, which can complicate the diagnosis and management of celiac disease.

26. What lifestyle changes can help manage SIBO?

Changes such as a balanced diet, stress management, regular exercise, and adequate hydration help improve intestinal motility and strengthen the immune system, supporting the treatment of SIBO.

27. Are there home tests to diagnose SIBO?

Although breath test kits can be performed at home, a health professional must interpret the results and make the final diagnosis.

28. Can SIBO affect the absorption of medications?

Yes, SIBO can alter the absorption of certain medications due to changes in intestinal pH and motility, which could affect their efficacy and levels in the body.

29. What type of specialist treats SIBO?

Gastroenterologists usually diagnose and treat SIBO, although they may also collaborate with dietitians and other health professionals.

30. What is the long-term prognosis for people with SIBO?

The prognosis varies depending on the underlying cause and response to treatment. With proper management, many people can control their symptoms and improve their quality of life. However, recurrence is possible and requires continued follow-up.

31. Can SIBO affect body weight?

Yes, SIBO can contribute to unintentional weight loss due to nutrient malabsorption and weight gain, as some people may experience changes in metabolism and fat storage.

32. Are there any long-term complications associated with SIBO?

If not adequately treated, SIBO can lead to complications such as nutritional deficiencies, damage to the intestinal lining, and an increased risk of developing inflammatory bowel conditions.

33. What role do digestive enzymes play?

Digestive enzymes help significantly improve digestion and nutrient absorption if SIBO has affected the natural enzyme production in the intestine.

34. How is SIBO related to chronic fatigue?

Nutrient malabsorption and systemic inflammation caused by SIBO can contribute to chronic fatigue. The body does not receive the nutrients needed to maintain energy and overall well-being.

35. Can SIBO cause skin changes?

Yes, SIBO can be related to skin problems such as acne, rosacea, eczema, and rashes due to inflammation, imbalance in gut microorganisms, and altered immune reaction.

36. Can SIBO affect liver function?

Yes, the toxins produced by the bacteria in the small intestine can overload the liver, the organ responsible for detoxification. This can affect its function and contribute to liver problems such as fatty liver.

37. Is it possible to prevent SIBO?
Preventing SIBO involves maintaining good digestive health through a balanced diet, managing stress, ensuring adequate intestinal motility, avoiding unnecessary antibiotics, and treating underlying conditions that may affect intestinal motility.

38. Can SIBO cause neurological symptoms?
Yes, SIBO can be associated with neurological symptoms such as brain fog, headaches, and concentration problems due to the connection between the gut and the brain.

39. Are there experimental treatments for SIBO?
Experimental treatments for SIBO may include specific probiotics, fecal microbiota transplants, and new drug therapies, although more research is needed to confirm their efficacy.

40. How does SIBO affect a person's daily life?
SIBO can significantly affect a person's quality of life by causing uncomfortable digestive symptoms and dietary restrictions and affecting emotional well-being due to the ongoing management of the disease.

41. What is the difference between SIBO and lactose intolerance?
Although both can cause similar digestive symptoms, such as bloating and diarrhea, SIBO is caused by an overgrowth of bacteria in the small intestine, while lactose intolerance is caused by a deficiency in the enzyme lactase, which is needed to digest the sugar in dairy products.

42. How does SIBO differ from other digestive conditions, such as irritable bowel syndrome (IBS)?
SIBO and IBS may share symptoms, but SIBO is specifically a bacterial growth in the small intestine, whereas IBS is a functional bowel disorder with causes that are not fully

understood. Breath tests are often used to differentiate between the two conditions.

43. Can stress trigger or worsen IBSB?
Yes, stress can affect intestinal motility, gastric acid production, gut microbiome balance, and immune function, which may contribute to the development or worsening of SIBO.

44. What is the role of prebiotics?
Prebiotics are fibers that feed beneficial bacteria in the gut. However, in the case of SIBO, they can exacerbate symptoms if not managed properly, so their use should be evaluated by a healthcare professional.

45. Does SIBO have any impact on cardiovascular health?
Although the direct impact of SIBO on cardiovascular health is still being investigated, chronic inflammation and malabsorption of essential nutrients such as omega-3 fatty acids could have adverse long-term effects on the cardiovascular system.

46. What type of diet is recommended?
The low-FODMAP diet is commonly recommended to reduce the symptoms of SIBO. It limits fermentable carbohydrates, which can feed the bacteria in the small intestine.

47. Can SIBO affect bone health?
Yes, people with SIBO can experience malabsorption of critical nutrients such as calcium and vitamin D, which are essential for bone health. This can increase the risk of osteoporosis.

48. How is it related to autoimmune diseases?
The disruption of the intestinal barrier and chronic inflammation caused by SIBO may activate inappropriate immune responses, contributing to the development or worsening of autoimmune diseases.

49. Is there any relationship between SIBO and food allergies?
Alterations in the intestinal mucosa caused by SIBO may increase intestinal permeability, contributing to sensitization

and the development of food allergies.

50. What recent research is being conducted on SIBO?
Current research explores new treatment options, such as the use of specific probiotics, the impact of the microbiome on SIBO, and its relationship to other health conditions.

51. Can SIBO be hereditary?
SIBO is not considered to be hereditary. However, genetic factors may influence intestinal motility or predisposition to certain conditions, increasing the risk of developing SIBO.

52. Are there gender differences in the prevalence of SIBO?
Some studies suggest that women may be more likely to develop SIBO than men, possibly due to hormonal and anatomical differences that affect intestinal motility.

53. How does the SCD or specific carbohydrate diet help treat SIBO?
The SCD diet helps by limiting complex carbohydrates that feed bacteria, thus reducing overgrowth and digestive symptoms.

54. What is the relationship between SIBO and gastro-esophageal reflux disease (GERD)?
Excess bacteria in the small intestine can produce gas that increases intra-abdominal pressure, contributing to acid reflux and GERD.

55. Can SIBO be a factor in the development of gluten intolerance?
Although not directly, SIBO can damage the intestinal mucosa and cause inflammation, exacerbating or triggering food intolerances, including gluten intolerance.

56. How is SIBO related to leaky gut syndrome?
SIBO can contribute to leaky gut syndrome by damaging the intestinal barrier and increasing inflammation. This allows toxins, undigested particles, and bacteria to enter the bloodstream and triggers inflammatory reactions.

57. What role does physical exercise play?

Regular exercise helps improve intestinal motility, which is beneficial in managing SIBO by promoting healthy intestinal transit and reducing the risk of bacterial growth.

58. Does SIBO affect the absorption of vitamins and minerals?

Yes, SIBO can affect the absorption of several vitamins and minerals, including vitamins B12, A, D, E, and K, as well as minerals such as iron and calcium, leading to nutritional deficiencies.

59. How do hormonal changes influence SIBO?

Hormonal changes, such as those that occur during the menstrual cycle, pregnancy, or menopause, can affect intestinal motility and, therefore, influence the development or exacerbation of SIBO.

60. Can SIBO cause respiratory problems?

Although uncommon, reflux and aspiration of gastric contents in people with SIBO may contribute to respiratory problems. If gases produced in the intestine rise into the esophagus and oral cavity, irritating the airways could also occur.

61. Can SIBO affect mental health?

Yes, SIBO can influence mental health. The connection between the gut and the brain is well-known, and gut inflammation or imbalances in the microbiome can contribute to symptoms of anxiety and depression.

62. Can SIBO be related to chronic fatigue syndrome (CFS)?

Yes, inflammation and malabsorption of essential nutrients in SIBO may contribute to chronic fatigue, a common symptom in CFS.

63. What role does serotonin play in SIBO?

Serotonin regulates intestinal motility. An imbalance in serotonin production can affect motility and contribute to the development of SIBO.

64. How is SIBO related to the skin and its conditions, such as acne or eczema?

Gut inflammation and bacterial imbalance can influence skin health, possibly exacerbating conditions such as acne or eczema.

65. What role do genetics play in predisposition to SIBO?

Although SIBO is not inherited, a genetic component may exist in predisposition to conditions that affect intestinal motility or the immune system.

66. Can SIBO increase the risk of infections in other parts of the body?

SIBO can affect the intestinal barrier and the immune system, potentially increasing the risk of systemic infections or infections in other body parts.

67. Can prolonged antibiotic treatment for SIBO cause antibiotic resistance?

Long-term antibiotic use can lead to antibiotic resistance; therefore, it is essential to follow medical guidelines and seek complementary alternatives.

68. Does SIBO affect thyroid function?

Due to the interaction between the immune system and intestinal health, SIBO may indirectly influence thyroid function, especially in people with autoimmune diseases such as Hashimoto's thyroiditis.

69. Can SIBO influence carbohydrate metabolism?

Bacterial overgrowth can interfere with the digestion and absorption of carbohydrates, affecting metabolism, blood sugar levels, and insulin response.

70. Can SIBO cause folic acid deficiencies?

Yes, although some bacteria produce folic acid, malabsorption in SIBO can lead to deficiencies of this essential vitamin.

71. Can SIBO cause problems in the endocrine system?

SIBO can indirectly influence the endocrine system by affecting the absorption of nutrients necessary for hormone production and altering the balance of the intestinal microbiome, which plays a role in hormone regulation.

72. How is SIBO related to polycystic ovary syndrome (PCOS)?
Although the direct connection is not fully established, the hormonal imbalance in PCOS may affect gut motility, increasing the risk of SIBO. In addition, chronic inflammation associated with SIBO may exacerbate PCOS symptoms.

73. Can SIBO influence blood sugar levels?
Yes, SIBO can affect carbohydrate digestion and absorption, leading to fluctuations in blood sugar levels and potentially contributing to spikes and crashes in glucose levels.

74. Can SIBO affect oral health?
Excess bacteria produce gases that can enter the oral cavity, leading to oral health problems such as bad breath or a change in taste.

75. Can SIBO be a factor in liver dysfunction?
SIBO can contribute to liver dysfunction by increasing the burden of toxins that the liver must process, especially if there is bacterial translocation (passage of bacteria from the gut) or endotoxemia (bacterial toxins in the blood).

76. Can SIBO cause fluid retention?
In some people with SIBO, intestinal inflammation and metabolic alterations can contribute to liquid retention.

77. Can SIBO cause joint problems?
Systemic inflammation caused by SIBO can contribute to joint problems or exacerbate existing inflammatory conditions in the joints.

78. What impact does SIBO have on fat absorption?
Excess bacteria can break down bile acids necessary for fat absorption, leading to fat malabsorption and symptoms such as fatty diarrhea.

79. Can SIBO cause changes in appetite?

Yes, some people with SIBO may experience loss of appetite due to digestive discomfort, while others may have an increased appetite in response to nutrient malabsorption.

80. How can SIBO be prevented after treatment?
To prevent the recurrence of SIBO, it is essential to address the underlying causes, follow a proper diet, maintain good intestinal motility, and, in some cases, use probiotics or maintenance treatment as directed by a healthcare professional.

81. How does SIBO affect the microbiota of the colon?
The movement of bacteria into the small intestine can alter the average balance of the colon's microbiome, affecting its function and health.

82. Can SIBO be related to fibromyalgia?
Some studies have found a higher prevalence of SIBO in people with fibromyalgia, suggesting a possible connection between the two conditions.

83. Can SIBO be related to migraines?
Some studies suggest that inflammation and the release of bacterial toxins in SIBO may be related to migraines in some people.

84. What role do bile acids play in SIBO?
Bile acids are essential for fat digestion. In SIBO, bacteria can break down bile acids, affecting fat digestion and absorption and causing diarrhea.

85. Can SIBO cause allergic skin reactions?
Although uncommon, SIBO can contribute to allergic reactions or skin rashes due to systemic inflammation and increased intestinal permeability.

86. Can SIBO be a factor in premenstrual syndrome (PMS)?
Although not directly related, SIBO can exacerbate PMS symptoms due to systemic inflammation and hormonal imbalance.

87. Can SIBO cause abdominal bloating?
Yes, bacteria in the small intestine ferment carbohydrates to produce gas, which can cause bloating and abdominal distention.

88. What impact does SIBO have on mineral absorption?
SIBO can affect the absorption of minerals such as iron, calcium, and magnesium, leading to nutritional deficiencies.

89. Can SIBO cause sleep problems?
Yes, uncomfortable digestive symptoms and systemic inflammation can interfere with sleep, causing insomnia or unrefreshing sleep.

90. Are there alternative therapies for the treatment of SIBO?
Many people find relief in alternative therapies such as acupuncture, phytotherapy, or functional medicine, among others.

91. Can SIBO cause changes in the intestinal rhythm, such as diarrhea or constipation?
SIBO can cause diarrhea and constipation depending on the predominant bacteria and their activity.

92. How is SIBO related to depression and anxiety?
The gut-brain axis can be affected by SIBO, and imbalances in the gut microbiome can influence the production of neurotransmitters, contributing to depression and anxiety.

93. Can SIBO cause alcohol intolerance?
Some people with SIBO report an increased sensitivity to alcohol, possibly due to altered gut flora and liver function.

94. Can it be related to eating disorders?
Some people with SIBO may develop excessive preoccupation with food and diet because of their symptoms, which may contribute to the development of eating disorders.

95. Can SIBO affect hormone balance in men?
Yes, as in women, SIBO can affect hormone balance in men by

influencing the absorption of nutrients necessary for hormone production.

96. Can SIBO cause vision problems?
Although uncommon, a deficiency of specific vitamins and nutrients due to SIBO may affect eye health and vision.

97. What role does fiber play in the management of SIBO?
Although fiber is essential for intestinal health, in the context of SIBO, inadequate fiber intake or certain types of fiber can exacerbate symptoms by being fermented by bacteria in the small intestine. Consult a health professional.

98. How does SIBO influence intestinal gas production?
SIBO can increase the production of gases such as hydrogen and methane, leading to symptoms such as bloating, flatulence, and abdominal discomfort.

99. Can SIBO have an impact on the mental health of children?
Yes, as in adults, SIBO in children can affect the gut-brain axis, potentially influencing their mood and behavior, contributing to anxiety problems and mood swings.

100. What is the role of probiotics?
Probiotics can help restore the balance of the gut microbiome. However, a healthcare professional should carefully evaluate their use in treating SIBO, as some strains may not be beneficial.

101. Can SIBO cause essential fatty acid deficiencies?
Yes, fat malabsorption in SIBO can lead to deficiencies of essential fatty acids, which are crucial for many bodily functions.

102. Are there specific supplements that can help?
Some supplements, such as those containing digestive enzymes, probiotics, zinc, glutamine, vitamin D, and specific prebiotics, support intestinal health and help manage SIBO.

103. Can SIBO affect oral health?

Nutrient malabsorption and bacterial growth can influence oral health, potentially increasing the risk of problems such as gingivitis or bad breath.

104. How is SIBO related to concentration problems?
Systemic inflammation and impaired absorption of essential nutrients can affect cognitive function, contributing to concentration and memory problems.

105. Is the treatment of SIBO permanent?
Treatment can reduce or eliminate bacterial overgrowth, but SIBO can recur if the underlying causes, such as intestinal motility problems or sphincter dysfunction, are not addressed.

106. What is the role of intestinal motility in SIBO?
Poor intestinal motility can allow bacteria to colonize the small intestine, contributing to the development of SIBO.

107. Can SIBO cause neurological symptoms?
Yes, some people with SIBO report neurological symptoms such as mental confusion or difficulty concentrating, possibly due to inflammation and bacterial toxin production.

108. What impact does SIBO have on the lymphatic system?
Inflammation and permeability of the intestine can affect the lymphatic system, which may contribute to fluid retention and swelling.

109. Can SIBO cause joint pain?
Although not directly causative, the systemic inflammation associated with SIBO can exacerbate joint pain or contribute to its development.

110. Are there natural treatments for SIBO?
Some natural treatments include antimicrobial herbs, such as oregano, garlic, and grapefruit seed extract.

111. How does SIBO influence iron absorption?
Malabsorption of nutrients in SIBO can cause iron deficiency, which could lead to anemia.

112. How does SIBO influence kidney health?

Although there is no direct relationship, systemic inflammation and electrolyte imbalances associated with SIBO can influence kidney function.

113. How does SIBO affect vitamin production by intestinal bacteria?

Although some intestinal bacteria produce vitamins such as vitamin K and some B-complex vitamins, SIBO can disrupt this process and contribute to deficiencies.

114. What is the impact of SIBO on cholesterol and blood lipids?

Fat malabsorption and altered lipid metabolism can affect cholesterol and other blood lipid levels.

115. Can SIBO be related to post-viral fatigue syndrome?

Some theories suggest that viral infections can alter intestinal motility, which could contribute to the development of SIBO and symptoms of chronic fatigue.

116. Can SIBO cause systemic inflammation?

Yes, bacterial translocation and toxin release can contribute to systemic inflammation, affecting multiple systems in the body.

117. Can SIBO influence thyroid hormone production?

Intestinal inflammation and malabsorption of nutrients essential for thyroid function can influence the production and regulation of thyroid hormones.

118. What impact does SIBO have on the mental health of older adults?

In older adults, SIBO can exacerbate mental health problems such as depression and anxiety and can also influence cognitive function.

119. Can SIBO cause sensitivity to cold or heat?

Although not a common symptom, hormonal and nutritional imbalances associated with SIBO may influence body temperature regulation.

120. Are there lifestyle changes that can help?
Yes, changes such as a healthy, balanced diet, stress management, regular exercise, and adequate rest are beneficial in managing SIBO.

121. Can SIBO affect heart health?
Although SIBO does not directly affect the heart, chronic inflam-mation and oxidative stress can contribute to long-term cardiovascular problems.

122. How is SIBO related to the enteric nervous system?
The enteric nervous system controls gastrointestinal function. Alterations in this system, such as reduced intestinal motility, may contribute to the development of SIBO.

123. Can SIBO cause changes in stool color?
Yes, SIBO can change stool color and consistency due to the malabsorption of fats and other nutrients.

124. Can SIBO cause vitamin A deficiencies?
Yes, malabsorption of fats in the stool can lead to deficiencies of fat-soluble vitamins, including vitamin A.

125. Can SIBO cause hair loss?
In people with SIBO, malabsorption of essential nutrients such as iron, zinc, and B vitamins can contribute to hair loss.

126. Can SIBO cause food sensitivities?
Yes, damage and inflammation in the small intestine can increase intestinal permeability, leading to food sensitivities.

127. Can SIBO influence the development of environ-mental allergies?
An imbalance of microorganisms in the gut and increased intestinal permeability may contribute to developing or exacerbating environmental allergies.

128. What impact does SIBO have on aging?
Chronic inflammation and malabsorption of nutrients can accelerate specific aging processes and affect overall health.

129. Can SIBO cause electrolyte imbalances?
Yes, chronic diarrhea and malabsorption can lead to imbalances in electrolytes such as sodium, potassium, and magnesium.

130. Are there complementary therapies that can help with SIBO?
Some complementary therapies, such as acupuncture, yoga, tai chi, and meditation, can help manage stress and improve overall well-being, which is beneficial for SIBO sufferers.

131. Can SIBO affect eye health?
Although uncommon, malabsorption of essential vitamins such as A and E could affect eye health.

132. How does SIBO influence protein metabolism?
SIBO can interfere with protein digestion and absorption, which could lead to deficiencies of essential amino acids and loss of muscle mass.

133. Can SIBO cause swelling in other parts of the body besides the abdomen?
Inflammation and fluid retention associated with SIBO may contribute to swelling in the extremities or other body areas.

134. How is SIBO related to lactose intolerance?
SIBO can affect lactose digestion by damaging the cells in the small intestine that produce lactase, the enzyme needed to digest lactose.

135. What role does stomach acid play?
Stomach acid helps kill bacteria that enter the digestive system with food. Low stomach acid levels can allow more bacteria to reach the small intestine, increasing the risk of SIBO.

SUGGESTED PRACTICAL PLAN

The treatment of SIBO requires a comprehensive approach that addresses the many factors necessary to restore gut health and alleviate associated symptoms. This method provides you with a clear and practical path to recovery. Let's dive in!

▸ **Identify the Possible Cause**: Uncovering the root causes of SIBO is a vital first step on your journey to recovery. Work to address, eliminate, or minimize the triggers that may be contributing to the condition's persistence. For a more in-depth understanding, be sure to consult the chapter titled "SIBO"–particularly the section "Causes of SIBO". This foundational step is critical for creating a solid framework for your healing process.

▸ **Nutrition**: A balanced and tailored diet is essential in managing SIBO. Certain foods and beverages help regenerate your gut system, while others can exacerbate symptoms. Mastering this distinction is key.
In the chapters "Foods That Transform" and "Juices and Smoothies," you'll find all the guidance you need, including more than 50 recipes crafted for your daily meals and an extensive assortment of juices and smoothies specifically designed for SIBO. Eating well is not only nourishing–it can also be delicious and comforting!

▸ **Supplements**: Nutritional supplements are fundamental for restoring intestinal balance and preparing your body for the subsequent stages. These supplements are designed to strengthen a weakened gut and effectively reduce inflammation. Be sure to follow the detailed guidelines in the chapter titled "Nutritional Supplements" and the section called "Supplements for SIBO: 9-Step Plan."
You can complete all nine steps by incorporating every

supplement suggested in the plan, or, if you prefer, you may focus on just the first four steps and then transition to medicinal plants in the fifth step. The decision is yours–set the pace of your process based on what feels most appropriate for you!

▸ **Medicinal Plants**: After completing the first four steps of the "Supplements for SIBO: 9-Step Plan," it's time to incorporate medicinal plants. In this fifth step, these plants act as a natural aid to effectively eliminate bacterial overgrowth and support the restoration of intestinal balance. This approach ensures your digestive system is well-prepared to maximize the benefits of herbal therapy.

You can find the recommended medicinal plants and herbal recipes in the chapter titled "Medicinal Plants," located in the section "Effective Plants for Managing SIBO," or in "Herbal Therapy Recipes." These natural and straightforward resources will seamlessly complement your recovery process and play a significant role in your overall well-being.

▸ **Medication**: If you're taking medications that you suspect may be worsening your symptoms or causing new issues, don't hesitate to consult your doctor. It may be necessary to adjust your treatment or modify the dosage to ensure that the medications do not interfere with your recovery process.

▸ **Lifestyle**: Your daily habits have a direct influence on the health of your digestive system. Engaging in activities like walking, dancing, or any form of regular physical exercise can stimulate intestinal motility–a key factor in improving SIBO symptoms. Choose activities you enjoy and make them a consistent part of your routine. Remember, movement is life–and it's also crucial for gut health!

▸ **Relaxation Techniques**: Stress is a silent enemy that can exacerbate SIBO symptoms. For this reason, incorporating stress management techniques into your routine is just as important as taking supplements or maintaining a proper diet. Practices like meditation, mindfulness, deep breathing, yoga, or tai chi can be powerful tools to help you relax, benefiting both your body and mind. Emotional well-being is an integral part of the healing process!

Remember: This book is designed to guide you step by step by providing the tools you need to restore your health and well-being. While the road to recovery may feel long, each small step you take matters and brings you closer to a better quality of life. You are not alone on this journey–every effort you make is an investment in your health!

Addressing Related Conditions

If you're managing other conditions alongside SIBO–such as diabetes, fibromyalgia, constipation, insomnia, anxiety, or menopause–it's important to remember that you are not alone. You may find it beneficial to explore my other books, which have been thoughtfully crafted to provide guidance, remedies, and practical strategies tailored to these specific challenges. These resources could offer valuable tools to support you on your journey toward better health and overall well-being.

- **Anxiety**. Foods, Supplements & Medicinal Plants
- **Diabetes**. Foods, Supplements & Medicinal Plants
- **Constipation**. Foods, Supplements & Medicinal Plants
- **Fibromyalgia**. Foods, Supplements & Medicinal Plants
- **Insomnia**. Foods, Supplements & Medicinal Plants
- **Menopause**. Foods, Supplements & Medicinal Plants

NUTRITIONAL SUPPLEMENTS

"Supplements are little allies that give us an extra boost on our way to optimal health"
(Dr. Mark Hyman)

Nutritional supplements have become a valuable ally in the pursuit of better health and an enhanced quality of life. These options–available in various user-friendly formats such as tablets, capsules, powders, or easily consumable liquids–are purposefully designed to complement your daily nutrition by delivering essential nutrients that can be challenging to obtain through regular meals alone. Packed with powerful components like vitamins, minerals, amino acids, antioxidants, and other bioactive compounds, these supplements are expertly formulated in precise proportions to meet the unique needs of every individual–even when the demands are high. Whether you're navigating restrictive diets, facing nutritional gaps, or coping with increased physical or mental demands, supplements can provide the extra support your body needs.

Beyond simply filling in nutritional gaps, supplements offer an array of tailored benefits to suit diverse lifestyles and health challenges. They can help boost energy, improve physical performance, support those managing fast-paced lives, and provide practical solutions for staying balanced and resilient. Their significance often becomes even more apparent during times of illness, specific health conditions, or chronic issues. In these situations, supplements do more than complement a diet –they can actively help restore altered functions, ease symptoms, and assist in more complex recovery processes. They serve as companions in the pursuit of health, helping you sustain and rebuild your vitality.

Effectively integrating supplements into your routine requires thoughtful use grounded in science and, when needed, professional guidance. By understanding their benefits and approaching them with care, supplements can evolve into powerful tools for improving your overall well-being in a sustainable and meaningful way. Remember–every step you take toward caring for your body is a step closer to feeling stronger, more energized, and more capable of facing life's challenges with confidence.

Take that step today. Your path to better health begins with small but impactful choices!

Essential Precautions

Understanding the risks associated with supplements is vital, as they can sometimes cause side effects, have contraindications, or interact with medications. It's important to thoroughly review the potential adverse effects detailed at the end of this chapter. Take a moment to assess your overall health and avoid any supplements that could conflict with the medications you're currently taking or exacerbate existing medical conditions. Prioritizing this step ensures a safer and more effective approach to improving your well-being.

Dosage, Usage and Benefits of the Supplements

The following provides a detailed summary of the key information on the dosage, usage instructions, and benefits of each recommended supplement, arranged alphabetically for your convenience:

Aloe Vera

▸ **Benefits**: Aloe vera helps reduce inflammation and promote digestive health in cases of SIBO.

▸ **Recommended Daily Dose**: The typical dose of aloe vera juice for digestive issues like SIBO ranges from 30 to 90 ml twice daily.

▸ **Dosage:** It is recommended that it be taken in the morning and evening, preferably before meals, to soothe the digestive tract and enhance the absorption of its properties.

Amylase

- **Benefits**: This digestive enzyme is beneficial for SIBO as it helps break down complex carbohydrates.

- **Recommended daily dose**: Generally between 2,000 to 5,000 FCC units per meal.

- **Dosage**: It is typically taken with meals, spreading the dose throughout the day to enhance carbohydrate digestion.

Berberine

Berberine is a natural compound traditionally used in Chinese medicine and is beneficial in addressing SIBO.

- **Benefits**: It possesses antimicrobial and anti-inflammatory properties that help reduce bacterial overgrowth in the small intestine, improve intestinal health, relieve inflammation, and alleviate digestive symptoms associated with SIBO.

- **Recommended daily dose**: The typical dose of berberine for SIBO is 500 to 1,500 mg, taken two or three times a day.

- **Dosage**: It may be taken in the morning, afternoon, and evening, preferably before meals, to better control digestive symptoms and enhance the compound's absorption.

Broad Spectrum Probiotics

- **Benefits**: Broad-spectrum probiotics contain a variety of beneficial bacterial strains that help restore the balance of the gut microbiota in individuals with SIBO. These probiotics contribute to improved gut health, strengthened immune function, and reduced inflammation in the gastrointestinal tract.

- **Recommended daily dose**: The recommended daily dosage may vary depending on strain concentration, symptom severity, and the manufacturer's recommendation. Generally, doses range from 10 to 50 billion CFU (colony-forming units) daily, emphasizing the importance of following product directions.

▸ **Dosage:** Broad-spectrum probiotics can be taken once or twice a day, preferably on an empty stomach or between meals, to enhance their survival in the digestive tract. Some individuals prefer morning intake, while others opt for evening consumption. Dosage and timing may vary according to the manufacturer's instructions and individual response, highlight-ing the necessity of adhering to specific recom-mendations.

Bromelain

Bromelain is a proteolytic enzyme found in pineapple that offers benefits in addressing SIBO.

▸ **Benefits:** Bromelain improves protein digestion, reduces inflammation in the gastrointestinal tract, and supports overall digestive function, which is advantageous for individuals with SIBO.

▸ **Recommended daily dose:** The typical dose of bromelain for SIBO is 500 to 1,000 mg, taken twice daily.

▸ **Dosage:** It can be taken in the morning and evening, preferably on an empty stomach or between meals, to enhance absorption.

Curcumin

▸ **Benefits:** Curcumin, an active compound in turmeric, possesses anti-inflammatory and antioxidant properties that aid in reducing inflammation and supporting digestive health.

▸ **Recommended daily dose:** The recommended daily dose of curcumin can vary but is generally between 500 to 1,500 mg per day.

▸ **Dosage:** It can be taken once or twice daily, preferably with meals to enhance absorption.

Ginger

▸ **Benefits:** Ginger is renowned for its ability to alleviate nausea, enhance digestion, and reduce inflammation in the gastrointestinal tract. For SIBO, ginger helps relieve digestive symptoms like bloating and gas.

‣ **Recommended daily dose**: The average daily dose varies but typically ranges from 1 to 3 grams of fresh ginger or 2 to 4 grams of dried ginger. For ginger supplements in capsule form, follow the manufacturer's instructions for dosage.

‣ **Dosage**: Ginger can be taken multiple times daily as needed to alleviate digestive symptoms. It can be consumed before or after meals, depending on individual preference and tolerance. Some individuals find it beneficial to take ginger before meals to aid digestion.

Glutamine

Glutamine is an amino acid that plays a crucial role in gut health and offers benefits in addressing SIBO.

‣ **Benefits**: It is known for its ability to repair and maintain the intestinal barrier, promote the health of intestinal cells, support immune function, and reduce gut inflammation.

‣ **Recommended daily dose**: The typical dose of glutamine for SIBO is 500 to 2,000 mg, taken two to three times daily.

‣ **Dosage**: Glutamine can be taken in the morning, afternoon, and evening, preferably on an empty stomach or between meals to enhance absorption.

GOS Prebiotics

‣ **Benefits**: Galactooligosaccharides (GOS) prebiotics benefit SIBO by promoting the growth of beneficial bacteria in the gut, enhancing gut health, and regulating gut microbiota. This helps alleviate symptoms associated with bacterial imbalance.

‣ **Recommended daily dose**: The recommended daily dose may vary depending on the product and concentration, so it is advisable to follow the manufacturer's instructions.

‣ **Dosage:** GOS prebiotics are typically taken once or twice daily, preferably with meals, to enhance their effectiveness and minimize potential gastrointestinal side effects. However, dosage and timing may vary according to the manufacturer's instructions and individual response, underscoring the importance of following the specific recommendations for each product.

Inulin

‣ **Benefits:** Inulin, a prebiotic fiber, fosters the growth of beneficial bacteria in the gut and enhances digestive health. In cases of SIBO, inulin aids in balancing gut flora and reducing symptoms associated with bacterial imbalance.

‣ **Recommended daily dose:** The dose of inulin for SIBO may vary based on individual tolerance. Generally, doses range from 5 to 10 grams per day.

‣ **Dosage:** It is typically taken once or twice daily, ideally before meals, to promote the growth of beneficial gut bacteria. Start with low doses and gradually increase to prevent gastrointestinal discomfort.

Iron

‣ **Benefits:** Iron is essential for red blood cell production and oxygen transport in the body. In cases of SIBO, where nutrient malabsorption is common, iron can help address iron deficiency anemia, a prevalent condition associated with this disorder.

‣ **Recommended daily dose:** The appropriate daily dose of iron for SIBO depends on the severity of the iron deficiency. Generally, doses range from 30 to 120 mg per day, but it is vital to consult your doctor to determine the suitable dose for your specific case.

‣ **Dosage:** Iron is typically taken once daily in the morning on an empty stomach or between meals to optimize absorption. Avoid consuming it with foods containing caffeine, calcium, or fiber, as these can hinder iron absorption. Taking it with food can help reduce gastrointestinal irritation if stomach upset occurs.

Magnesium

Magnesium is an essential mineral vital for numerous body functions, including the proper functioning of the digestive system.

▸ **Benefits**: It helps relieve constipation, a common symptom in individuals with SIBO, by promoting bowel regularity and enhancing gastrointestinal motility. Additionally, it relaxes the intestinal muscles, which is advantageous for those with SIBO.

▸ **Recommended daily dose**: The usual dosage for SIBO is typically between 200 and 400 mg daily.

▸ **Dosage**: Magnesium can be taken in the morning, afternoon, or evening, preferably on an empty stomach or between meals. However, certain forms of magnesium, like magnesium citrate, can be taken with meals.

N-acetylcysteine (NAC)

N-acetylcysteine (NAC) is a compound utilized in medicine for its antioxidant properties and capacity to elevate glutathione levels in the body.

▸ **Benefits**: It possesses antioxidant properties that help reduce inflammation in the gut, promote detoxification, and safeguard intestinal cells.

▸ **Recommended daily dose**: The typical dose of NAC for SIBO is 600 to 1,200 mg twice daily.

▸ **Dosage**: It can be taken in the morning and evening, preferably on an empty stomach or between meals, to enhance absorption.

Omega-3

▸ **Benefits**: Omega-3 fatty acids, such as EPA and DHA, have anti-inflammatory properties that are beneficial for SIBO by assisting in reducing gut inflammation and supporting the health of the gut lining.

▸ **Recommended daily dose**: The recommended dose varies, but 250-500 mg of EPA and DHA combined is typically advised to maintain overall good health.

▸ **Dosage**: Omega-3 can be taken at any time of the day, preferably with food to enhance absorption. Some prefer taking it in the morning, while others prefer the evening. There is no strict rule on when to take it, but consistency with the recommended daily dose is essential.

Oregano Oil

Due to its antimicrobial properties, oregano oil is a popular supplement for addressing SIBO.

▸ **Benefits:** It helps reduce bacterial overgrowth in the small intestine, relieves digestive symptoms, and promotes overall intestinal health.

▸ **Recommended Daily Dose:** The typical dose of oregano oil for SIBO is 200-500 mg, taken twice daily.

▸ **Dosage:** It can be taken in the morning and evening, preferably with meals to aid absorption.

Papain

Papain is a proteolytic enzyme found in papaya that offers benefits for SIBO.

▸ **Benefits:** It aids in improving protein digestion, reducing inflammation in the gastrointestinal tract, relieving bloating and gas, and supporting overall digestive function, which is advantageous for people dealing with SIBO.

▸ **Recommended daily dose:** The typical dose of papain for SIBO is 500 to 1,000 mg, taken twice daily.

‣ **Dosage**: It can be taken in the morning and evening, preferably on an empty stomach or between meals, to enhance absorption.

Prebiotics FOS

‣ **Benefits**: Prebiotics such as fructooligosaccharides (FOS) offer benefits for SIBO by promoting the growth of beneficial bacteria in the gut, enhancing the diversity of the gut microbiota, and helping to balance the bacterial flora. This, in turn, helps alleviate symptoms associated with bacterial imbalance.

‣ **Recommended daily dose**: The recommended daily dose may vary depending on the product and concentration, but it typically ranges from 2 to 5 grams per day. It is advisable to follow the manufacturer's instructions.

‣ **Dosage**: FOS prebiotics are generally taken once or twice daily, preferably with meals, to improve absorption and minimize potential gastrointestinal side effects. However, dosage and timing may vary according to the manufacturer's instructions and individual response, so it is crucial to adhere to the specific recommendations for each product.

Selenium

‣ **Benefits**: Selenium is a crucial antioxidant that aids in protecting cells from oxidative damage and maintaining immune system health. In the context of SIBO, selenium has been found to have positive effects on gut health by supporting immune function and reducing inflammation, thereby improving symptoms.

‣ **Recommended daily dose**: The recommended daily allowance of selenium varies depending on age, sex, and individual needs. Generally, the recommended daily amount for adults is approximately 55 micrograms.

‣ **Dosage**: Selenium supplementation is typically taken once daily, preferably with a meal to enhance absorption. There is no specific time to take selenium, so it can be consumed anytime.

Turmeric

Turmeric is a spice with anti-inflammatory and antioxidant properties. It is traditionally used in Ayurvedic medicine and is beneficial in treating SIBO.

‣ **Benefits**: It helps reduce gut inflammation, alleviate digestive symptoms, and support liver function, which is advantageous for individuals with SIBO.

‣ **Recommended daily dose**: The typical dose of turmeric in supplement form for SIBO is 500 to 1,500 mg, taken twice daily.

‣ **Dosage**: It can be taken in the morning and evening, preferably with meals to enhance the absorption.

Vitamin B12

Vitamin B12 is essential for forming red blood cells, properly functioning the nervous system, and macronutrient metabolism.

‣ **Benefits**: Vitamin B12 deficiency is common in individuals with SIBO, as bacteria in the small intestine can hinder the proper absorption of this vitamin. Vitamin B12 supplementation helps correct this deficiency and improves associated symptoms such as fatigue, weakness, and neurological problems.

‣ **Recommended daily dose**: The typical dose of vitamin B12 for SIBO varies but is generally recommended to be between 1,000 to 2,000 mcg per day, depending on the severity of the deficiency.

‣ **Dosage**: It can be taken in the morning, afternoon, or evening, preferably on an empty stomach or between meals. Some forms of vitamin B12 are better absorbed with food, so following the manufacturer's directions is essential.

Vitamin C

▸ **Benefits:** Vitamin C, also known as ascorbic acid, is a vital antioxidant that plays a crucial role in immune system health and antioxidant function in the body. In the context of SIBO, vitamin C helps strengthen the immune system, reduce inflammation, and support digestive system health, which is beneficial for individuals with SIBO.

▸ **Recommended daily dose:** In cases of SIBO, the recommended daily dose of vitamin C is 500 to 1,500 milligrams.

▸ **Dosage:** Vitamin C can be taken once or twice daily, preferably with meals to enhance absorption.

Vitamin D

Vitamin D regulates the body's immune system, bone health, and cellular function. In the context of SIBO, vitamin D deficiency may be associated with gastrointestinal disorders and imbalances in the gut microbiota.

▸ **Benefits:** Vitamin D is vital in modulating the immune response and gut health, which benefits people with SIBO. It has been suggested that vitamin D deficiency may be associated with an increased risk of developing SIBO and that supplementation helps to improve related symptoms.

▸ **Recommended daily dose:** The typical dose of vitamin D for SIBO varies, but it is generally recommended to be between 1,000 and 5,000 IU per day, depending on vitamin D blood levels.

▸ **Dosage:** It can be taken at any time of the day, preferably with a meal containing healthy fats to improve absorption. Some people prefer to take it in the morning to ensure they remember.

Zinc

Zinc is an essential mineral that is crucial for numerous bodily functions, including immune health, wound healing, and gastrointestinal function.

▸ **Benefits:** Zinc plays a vital role in immune function and intestinal barrier integrity, which benefits people with SIBO. Zinc deficiency has been associated with digestive problems and can worsen SIBO symptoms, so zinc supplementation is desirable and valuable.

‣ **Recommended daily dose:** The typical dose of zinc for SIBO varies, but it is generally recommended between 15 and 30 mg per day, depending on individual needs and the presence of zinc deficiency.

‣ **Dosage:** It can be taken any time of the day, preferably on an empty stomach or between meals, to improve absorption. Some people prefer to take it in the morning or evening to make it easier to incorporate into their daily routine.

Supplements for SIBO: A 9-Step Plan

SIBO treatment can be enhanced through the use of targeted supplements that not only help eliminate harmful bacteria but also support comprehensive gut recovery. While certain supplements may be used individually based on your specific needs, the most effective results for treating SIBO are achieved by following a structured and progressive plan, such as the one outlined below.

This approach goes beyond merely eradicating bacteria. It focuses on healing and strengthening your gut, restoring microbiota balance, and minimizing the likelihood of future relapses.

By following this step-by-step plan, you can effectively address each phase of the recovery process, paving the way for more sustainable and long-lasting improvements in your digestive health.

How does this approach work?

‣ First, we eliminate the problem: We target and reduce harmful bacteria using specific antimicrobials.
‣ Next, we repair the damage: We heal the intestinal lining, address nutritional deficiencies, and reduce inflammation.

▸ Then, we strengthen and stabilize: We provide antioxidant support, rebalance the microbiota, and enhance your immune system.

▸ Finally, we optimize digestion: We ensure your gut functions effectively and sustainably over the long term.

SIBO Treatment Plan (Step by Step)

This is a straightforward and progressive plan. You simply need to select one supplement per category based on the recommendations provided for each stage.

Important: Always review the potential adverse effects in the section titled "Side Effects, Contraindications, and Interactions" within this chapter to ensure you choose the safest and most suitable supplement for your specific needs.

▸ **Step 1: Antimicrobial Treatment**
  ▸ Goal: Eliminate the bacteria responsible for SIBO.
  ▸ Supplements: Berberine, oregano oil, or N-acetylcysteine (choose only one).
  ▸ Duration: 5 weeks.
  ▸ Tip: Follow a healthy diet to support this process; refer to the chapter "Foods That Transform".

▸ **Step 2: Enhance Intestinal Motility**
  ▸ Goal: Prevent the re-accumulation of eliminated bacteria.
  ▸ Supplements: Ginger, magnesium, or aloe vera (choose only one).
  ▸ Duration: 4 weeks.
  ▸ Tip: Stay hydrated, engage in regular exercise, and follow a digestion-friendly diet.

▸ **Step 3: Heal the Intestinal Mucosa**
  ▸ Goal: Repair damage to the intestinal barrier for better function.
  ▸ Supplements: Glutamine, zinc, or turmeric. (Choose only one)
  ▸ Duration: 5 weeks.

▸ **Step 4: Correct Nutritional Deficiencies**
  ▸ Goal: Restore nutrients lost due to SIBO.

- Supplements: Take only what you need according to your blood tests (e.g., Vitamin B12, iron, folate, Vitamin D, zinc, or magnesium).
- Duration: Depends on your needs (average: 8 weeks).
- Tip: Repeat blood tests every 6-7 weeks to monitor deficiency correction.

Step 5: Antioxidant Support and Cellular Recovery
- Goal: Repair cellular damage and reduce oxidative stress.
- Supplements: Vitamin C, zinc, or selenium. (Choose only one)
- Duration: 4-6 weeks.

Step 6: Reduce Intestinal Inflammation
- Goal: Soothe and protect the intestines.
- Supplements: Omega-3 or turmeric. (Choose only one)
- Duration: 6 weeks.
- Tip: Combine this step with a balanced diet and stress management.

Step 7: Rebalance Gut Microbiota
- Goal: Restore the balance of beneficial bacteria.
- Action: Take broad-spectrum probiotics along with one prebiotic (choose from inulin, FOS, or GOS).
- Duration: 6 weeks.
- Tip: Ensure the gut is well-repaired and has minimal inflammation before starting this step.

Step 8: Strengthen the Immune System
- Supplements: Vitamin D, glutathione, or turmeric. (Choose only one)
- Duration: 4-6 weeks.
- Tip: This step is important once your gut is balanced.

Step 9: Final Digestive Support
- Goal: Maintain long-term digestive health.
- Action: Use combinations like amylase + bromelain or papain to facilitate digestion.
- Duration: Based on your needs (minimum: 4 weeks).
- Tip: These enzymes will improve nutrient absorption and help you feel lighter.

Final Note for Chronic or Severe Cases

If your SIBO is chronic or you have significant intestinal damage:

‣ Extend Step 1 (antimicrobials) to 6 weeks under medical supervision.

‣ Intestinal motility may require long-term supplementation if it remains slow.

‣ Intestinal mucosa repair may take up to 8 weeks in severe cases.

‣ Microbiota rebalancing may need to be extended to 8-12 weeks to restore balance.

You may consult a specialized doctor to customize this plan according to your specific needs. Every body is unique, and proper follow-up care enhances outcomes. Best of luck with your recovery!

Side Effects, Contraindications, and Interactions

Outlined below is essential information regarding the potential side effects, contraindications, and interactions of the recommended supplements. It is strongly advised to review this carefully before beginning their use to ensure safe and responsible consumption.

Aloe vera

‣ **Side effects**: Aloe vera may lead to gastrointestinal irritation, including diarrhea and cramps. Some individuals may experience skin allergies, such as redness or itching. In high doses, aloe vera can act as a laxative and cause electrolyte imbalances.

‣ **Contraindications**: Aloe vera is not advisable during pregnancy as it may stimulate uterine contractions. Individuals with kidney or heart conditions should refrain from using it, as should those with known allergies.

‣ **Interactions**: Aloe vera may interact with diuretics and diabetes drugs, potentially intensifying their effects. It could also interact with heart medications, such as digoxin. To prevent potential adverse interactions, consult a healthcare provider or pharmacist before combining aloe vera with drugs.

Amylase

‣ **Side effects**: Some individuals may experience stomach upset, nausea, and diarrhea.

‣ **Contraindications**: Individuals with known allergies to amylase should refrain from consumption.

‣ **Interactions**: There are no significant drug interactions reported to date.

Berberine

‣ **Side effects**: In certain cases, individuals may encounter stomach upset, diarrhea, constipation, and nausea.

‣ **Contraindications**: Berberine may not be suitable for pregnant or lactating women, individuals allergic to plants of the Berberidaceae family, and those with severe liver or kidney disease.

‣ **Interactions**: Berberine has the potential to interact with medications that impact blood glucose levels, such as insulin or oral hypoglycemic agents, and certain drugs affecting liver metabolism. It is essential to consult your doctor pharmacist before use, especially if you are taking medication.

Broad-spectrum probiotics

‣ **Side effects**: Some individuals may experience mild side effects, such as gas, abdominal bloating, or gastrointestinal discomfort.

‣ **Contraindications**: Avoid them in case of compromised immune systems or severe health conditions.

‣ **Interactions**: No significant drug interactions have been identified at this time.

Bromelain

‣ **Side effects**: Some individuals may experience stomach upset, diarrhea, skin allergies, and, in sensitive cases, allergic reactions.

‣ **Contraindications**: Bromelain, which is derived from pineapple, is contraindicated for individuals allergic to tropical pineapple. Caution should also be exercised in individuals with coagulation disorders and stomach ulcers.

‣ **Interactions**: It may interact with certain medications, such as anticoagulants, antiplatelet drugs, and certain antibiotics. Consult with your healthcare provider or pharmacist if you are undergoing any pharmacological treatment.

Curcumin

‣ **Side effects**: High doses may lead to stomach upset, nausea, or diarrhea in some individuals.

‣ **Contraindications**: Curcumin is not recommended in cases of gallstones or individuals with biliary obstruction.

‣ **Interactions**: Curcumin may interact with anticoagulants, antiplatelets, and diabetes medications. Please consult a doctor or pharmacist before combining it with other drugs.

Ginger

‣ **Side effects**: High doses may lead to heartburn, diarrhea, or gastrointestinal irritation in specific individuals.

‣ **Contraindications**: Avoid individuals taking anticoagulant drugs or those with gallstones.

‣ **Interactions**: Ginger may interact with anticoagulant drugs, antiplatelet drugs, and blood pressure medications. Consult a healthcare professional before combining ginger with other medicines.

Glutamine

‣ **Side effects**: Some individuals may experience stomach

upset, bloating, headaches, and, in certain instances, muscle or joint issues.

‣ **Contraindications**: Glutamine is not recommended for individuals with severe kidney disease, liver disorders, seizure disorders, or those allergic to the supplement.

‣ **Interactions**: Glutamine may interact with certain medications, such as gamma-aminobutyric acid (GABA) absorption inhibitors and chemotherapy drugs. To prevent potential interactions, it is crucial to consult a healthcare professional before combining glutamine with medications.

GOS prebiotics

‣ **Side effects**: High doses may result in gas, bloating, and abdominal discomfort in some individuals.

‣ **Contraindications**: Avoid in individuals with intolerance to GOS or chronic gastrointestinal issues.

‣ **Interactions**: No significant drug interactions have been reported to date.

Inulin

‣ **Side effects**: Inulin may lead to flatulence, abdominal bloating, and gastrointestinal discomfort in some individuals.

‣ **Contraindications**: Individuals with inulin intolerance should refrain from consumption.

‣ **Interactions**: There are no significant drug interactions reported to date with inulin.

Iron

‣ **Side effects**: Possible side effects may include stomach upset, nausea, constipation, or dark stools.

‣ **Contraindications**: Iron supplementation should be avoided by individuals with iron overload, liver disease, or anemia unrelated to iron deficiency.

▸ **Interactions**: Iron may reduce the absorption of specific medications, such as antibiotics and thyroid medications. It may also interact with calcium or zinc supplements, decreasing iron absorption. Consultation with a healthcare provider or pharmacist before combining iron supplements with other drugs is recommended.

Magnesium

▸ **Side effects**: Some individuals may experience stomach upset, diarrhea, nausea, vomiting, and in high doses, it can act as a laxative.

▸ **Contraindications**: Not suitable for individuals with severe renal insufficiency, myasthenia gravis, Addison's disease, or those taking specific medications like diuretics or antibiotics.

▸ **Interactions**: Magnesium may interact with medications such as antibiotics, bisphosphonates, diuretics, and blood pressure medications.

N-acetylcysteine

▸ **Side effects**: Some individuals may experience mild side effects such as nausea, vomiting, diarrhea, headache, or upset stomach.

▸ **Contraindications**: Avoid use in individuals allergic to N-acetylcysteine or with a history of gastric ulcers.

▸ **Interactions**: N-acetylcysteine may interact with drugs like nitroglycerin, carbamazepine, and nitrofurantoin. Consult a healthcare professional before combining NAC with medications.

Omega-3

▸ **Side effects**: Some individuals may experience mild side effects, such as a fishy taste, fishy belching, bad breath, nausea, or diarrhea.

▸ **Contraindications:** To be avoided by individuals allergic to shellfish or fish and those with blood clotting disorders.

▸ **Interactions:** Omega-3 may interact with anticoagulants, antiplatelet, and blood pressure medications. Please consult your doctor before combining it with medications.

Oregano oil

▸ **Side effects:** When topically applied in high concentrations, potential side effects may include stomach upset, nausea, vomiting, skin allergies, and skin irritation.

▸ **Contraindications:** Oregano oil is not recommended for pregnant women, individuals with allergies to the mint family, and young children. Due to its potential impact on blood clotting, caution should also be exercised in individuals with bleeding disorders and before surgical procedures.

▸ **Interactions:** There is a possibility of interactions with medications that affect blood clotting, such as anticoagulants and drugs used to regulate blood sugar levels.

Papain

▸ **Side effects:** It may cause stomach upset, diarrhea, nausea, and sometimes mouth or throat irritation in specific individuals.

▸ **Contraindications:** If you are allergic to papaya, avoid using papain, as it is derived from the papaya fruit. Caution should be exercised in individuals with stomach ulcers or taking anticoagulant medication.

▸ **Interactions:** Papain may interact with medications such as anticoagulants and antiplatelet medications, potentially enhancing their effects.

Prebiotics FOS

▸ **Side effects:** High doses may lead to gas, bloating, and gastrointestinal discomfort.

‣ **Contraindications**: Avoid it in people with intolerance to FOS or irritable bowel syndrome.

‣ **Interactions**: No significant drug interactions are known at this time.

Selenium

‣ **Side effects**: High doses of selenium can lead to gastro-intestinal problems (nausea, vomiting, diarrhea), fatigue, hair loss, skin irritation, and neurological issues.

‣ **Contraindications**: This product should be avoided by individuals allergic to selenium, those with a history of kidney or liver disease, and pregnant or breastfeeding women.

‣ **Interactions**: It may interact with certain medications like blood thinners, thyroid medications, blood pressure medications, and some chemotherapeutics. Consult a healthcare provider before combining selenium with other medicines.

Turmeric

‣ **Side effects**: Stomach upset, heartburn, diarrhea, and, in rare instances, skin allergies may occur in some cases.

‣ **Contraindications**: Turmeric may not be suitable in large quantities for individuals with gallstones, bile duct obstruction, stomach ulcers, or known allergies to turmeric.

‣ **Interactions**: It may interact with certain medications, such as anticoagulants, antiplatelet drugs, heartburn relief medications, and some diabetes medications.

Vitamin B12

‣ **Side effects**: Vitamin B12 is considered safe and does not typically cause side effects in regular doses. However, very high doses can result in side effects like nervousness, anxiety, headache, nausea, and reddening of the skin.

‣ **Contraindications**: Generally safe for most individuals, but may not be suitable for those with a vitamin B12 allergy, severe kidney or liver disease, or specific cancers.

‣ **Interactions**: Vitamin B12 may interact with certain medications such as proton pump inhibitors, aminoglycoside antibiotics, metformin, and oral contraceptives. It may also interact with supplements like folic acid. Consult a healthcare professional before taking vitamin B12 supplements if you are on medication.

Vitamin C

‣ **Side effects**: High doses may lead to stomach upset, diarrhea, or kidney stones in some individuals.

‣ **Contraindications**: Avoid in case of kidney stones, hemochromatosis (iron accumulation), or severe kidney disease.

‣ **Interactions**: Vitamin C may interact with medications like blood thinners, ACE inhibitors, chemotherapy, and certain blood pressure medications. Consult a healthcare provider before combining vitamin C with drugs.

Vitamin D

‣ **Side effects**: Generally safe in adequate amounts, but very high doses can result in side effects such as nausea, vomiting, weakness, confusion, loss of appetite, and, in severe cases, toxicity.

‣ **Contraindications**: It is not recommended for individuals with high blood calcium levels, hypervitaminosis D, severe kidney or liver disease, sarcoidosis, or specific bone metabolism disorders.

‣ **Interactions**: Vitamin D may interact with medications like glucocorticoids, anticonvulsants, anticoagulants, and high blood pressure medications. Consult a healthcare professional if you are taking any medications.

Zinc

‣ **Side effects:** This may lead to stomach upset, nausea, vomiting, and diarrhea in some individuals.

‣ **Contraindications:** Zinc is unsuitable for individuals with severe kidney or liver disease or zinc allergies.

‣ **Interactions:** Zinc may interact with medications such as antibiotics, diuretics, oral contraceptives, and osteoporosis medications. High doses of zinc can impact the absorption of iron and calcium.

FOODS THAT TRANSFORM

*"We are what we eat. Healthy eating is the first step towards a complete
and harmonious life" (Ann Wigmore)*

Throughout history, our diet has undergone profoundly radical changes, sharply diverging from the habits of our ancestors. Millions of years ago, early humans shaped their diet around what they could gather or hunt, relying on fresh and raw foods provided by their environment. The emergence of agriculture and livestock farming marked the beginning of a new era of human nutrition, further accelerated by the Industrial Revolution. However, it is important to recognize that while our dietary habits have evolved drastically, our genetics have remained virtually unchanged.

Over time, foods such as dairy products, grains, refined sugars, and vegetable oils were introduced, alongside the rise of intensive meat production. These innovations have made meals more accessible and convenient, yet they have also led to significant changes in nutritional composition. Furthermore, advances in food preservation and culinary techniques gave rise to new methods of storage and preparation, which inevitably impacted food quality.

In recent years, an alarming trend has surfaced: modern diets have become dominated by ultra-processed foods, contributing to the widespread increase in chronic illnesses. Conditions such as obesity, type 2 diabetes, hypertension, and a variety of cardiovascular and digestive disorders have all been closely linked to this dietary shift. Why is this happening? Primarily because ultra-processed foods are heavily laden with refined carbohydrates, unhealthy fats, added sugars, chemical additives, and low-quality vegetable oils. Even meats and other animal products from intensive farming systems are often filled with substances harmful to health. These processed foods have largely replaced traditional diets, which were built on fresh and natural ingredients, disrupting the equilibrium that once fostered optimal well-being among our ancestors.

Nonetheless, there is hope for reversing this trend: small yet thoughtful changes to our eating habits can have a significant impact on our health. Returning to a balanced, nutrient-rich way of eating, centered on fresh, whole foods, is essential for establishing a strong foundation for wellness. Integrating fruits, vegetables, root vegetables, legumes, nuts, and seeds into the diet is a powerful step toward revitalizing the way we nourish ourselves. Despite this, one major challenge persists: the consumption of these natural, unprocessed foods remains astonishingly low in many parts of the world.

Choosing a lifestyle rooted in mindful eating not only helps prevent diseases associated with poor dietary habits but also rejuvenates the body and mind. By prioritizing real, wholesome foods and cutting back on ultra-processed options, we can cultivate a healthier, more balanced, and fulfilling life. Now is the time to rediscover the transformative power of a healthy diet–not as a form of restriction, but as an act of self-care. Your health deserves that commitment!

Throughout history, our diet has undergone profoundly radical changes, sharply diverging from the habits of our ancestors. Millions of years ago, early humans shaped their diet around what they could gather or hunt, relying on fresh and raw foods provided by their environment. The emergence of agriculture and livestock farming marked the beginning of a new era of human nutrition, further accelerated by the Industrial Revolution. However, it is important to recognize that while our dietary habits have evolved drastically, our genetics have remained virtually unchanged.

Over time, foods such as dairy products, grains, refined sugars, and vegetable oils were introduced, alongside the rise of intensive meat production. These innovations have made meals more accessible and convenient, yet they have also led to significant changes in nutritional composition. Furthermore, advances in food preservation and culinary techniques gave rise to new methods of storage and preparation, which inevitably impacted food quality.

In recent years, an alarming trend has surfaced: modern diets have become dominated by ultra-processed foods, contributing to the widespread increase in chronic illnesses. Conditions such as obesity, type 2 diabetes, hypertension, and a variety of cardiovascular and digestive disorders have all been closely linked to this dietary shift. Why is this happening? Primarily because ultra-processed foods are heavily laden with refined carbohydrates, unhealthy fats, added sugars, chemical additives, and low-quality vegetable oils. Even meats and other animal products from intensive farming systems are often filled with substances harmful to health. These processed foods have largely replaced traditional diets, which were built on fresh and natural ingredients, disrupting the equilibrium that once fostered optimal well-being among our ancestors.

Nonetheless, there is hope for reversing this trend: small yet thoughtful changes to our eating habits can have a significant impact on our health. Returning to a balanced, nutrient-rich way of eating, centered on fresh, whole foods, is essential for establishing a strong foundation for wellness. Integrating fruits, vegetables, root vegetables, legumes, nuts, and seeds into the diet is a powerful step toward revitalizing the way we nourish ourselves. Despite this, one major challenge persists: the consumption of these natural, unprocessed foods remains astonishingly low in many parts of the world.

Choosing a lifestyle rooted in mindful eating not only helps prevent diseases associated with poor dietary habits but also rejuvenates the body and mind. By prioritizing real, wholesome foods and cutting back on ultra-processed options, we can cultivate a healthier, more balanced, and fulfilling life. Now is the time to rediscover the transformative power of a healthy diet–not as a form of restriction, but as an act of self-care. Your health deserves that commitment!

Understanding the Link Between Nutrition and Health

How often have you asked yourself if what you eat truly supports your well-being? The relationship between nutrition and health is far deeper than we commonly realize. Understanding which foods promote wellness and which ones to avoid, tailored to your specific needs, is a powerful step toward improving your quality of life. This isn't a new concept; it has been examined and revered for centuries. Since ancient times, cultures around the world have recognized the therapeutic value of nutrition as a means to heal, strengthen, and sustain the body, leaving us a profound legacy of wisdom.

Traditional medical systems–such as Traditional Chinese Medicine, the practices of ancient Egypt, Greece, and Rome, Ayurveda in India, and indigenous healing methods across the Americas–delved into the restorative potential of natural foods. These practices emphasized the idea that food does much more than nourish; it can protect, alleviate discomfort, and even heal the body.

For many years, these age-old principles were often dismissed by conventional medicine as unscientific. Yet, modern research has gradually confirmed what our ancestors intuitively understood: the foods we eat directly affect not only our physical health but also our emotional well-being. Today, scientific studies continue to uncover compounds in food with therapeutic properties that help prevent diseases, reduce symptoms, and promote overall health.

Researchers have spent decades analyzing how certain foods strengthen the body and protect against chronic illnesses, identifying dietary patterns in populations with low disease rates that differ significantly from those in less healthy communities. These studies reveal the decisive role specific nutrients play in promoting vitality and longevity, with certain foods offering unique benefits such as anti-inflammatory properties to manage joint pain and chronic discomfort, antimicrobial effects to bolster immune defenses, anticoagulant actions to support cardiovascular health, antihypertensive abilities to regulate blood pressure, and mood-enhancing compounds that alleviate anxiety while fostering emotional resilience.

What you choose to eat influences not only your daily energy but also your capacity to recover, fend off illness, and pursue a fulfilling life. On the flip side, a poor diet or reliance on unhealthy foods can exacerbate health problems, intensify symptoms, and undermine overall well-being.

The encouraging part? Every day offers the chance to make dietary choices that lead to better health. While external factors like pollution or environmental changes may remain out of your control, your diet is a fundamental tool for self-care. Each ingredient on your plate carries the potential to positively impact both your physical and mental health.

Learning which foods are best for your unique needs–and understanding which ones may harm your health–can empower you to find balance and achieve a healthier, more vibrant lifestyle. Nutrition, humanity's earliest form of medicine, is not just a pathway to wellness but also a connection to our roots, equipping us for a future filled with possibilities.

I invite you to explore how nutrition can become your strongest ally in easing ailments, building resilience, and fostering happiness. Are you ready to embrace this journey of discovery and transformation? Your well-being is within your control, and every meal is a chance to create a life of greater health and vitality.

Start today: Nourish your body, refresh your mind, and live fully. How often have you asked yourself if what you eat truly supports your well-being? The relationship between nutrition and health is far deeper than we commonly realize. Understanding which foods promote wellness and which ones to avoid, tailored to your specific needs, is a powerful step toward improving your quality of life. This isn't a new concept; it has been examined and revered for centuries. Since ancient times, cultures around the world have recognized the therapeutic value of nutrition as a means to heal, strengthen, and sustain the body, leaving us a profound legacy of wisdom.

Traditional medical systems–such as Traditional Chinese Medicine, the practices of ancient Egypt, Greece, and Rome, Ayurveda in India, and indigenous healing methods across the Americas–delved into the restorative potential of natural foods. These practices emphasized the idea that food does much more than nourish; it can protect, alleviate discomfort, and even heal the body.

For many years, these age-old principles were often dismissed by conventional medicine as unscientific. Yet, modern research has gradually confirmed what our ancestors intuitively understood: the foods we eat directly affect not only our physical health but also our emotional well-being. Today, scientific studies continue to uncover compounds in food with therapeutic properties that help prevent diseases, reduce symptoms, and promote overall health.

Researchers have spent decades analyzing how certain foods strengthen the body and protect against chronic illnesses, identifying dietary patterns in populations with low disease rates that differ significantly from those in less healthy communities. These studies reveal the decisive role specific nutrients play in promoting vitality and longevity, with certain foods offering unique benefits such as anti-inflammatory properties to manage joint pain and chronic discomfort, antimicrobial effects to bolster immune defenses, anticoagulant actions to support cardiovascular health, antihypertensive abilities to regulate blood pressure, and mood-enhancing compounds that alleviate anxiety while fostering emotional resilience.

What you choose to eat influences not only your daily energy but also your capacity to recover, fend off illness, and pursue a fulfilling life. On the flip side, a poor diet or reliance on unhealthy foods can exacerbate health problems, intensify symptoms, and undermine overall well-being.

The encouraging part? Every day offers the chance to make

dietary choices that lead to better health. While external factors like pollution or environmental changes may remain out of your control, your diet is a fundamental tool for self-care. Each ingredient on your plate carries the potential to positively impact both your physical and mental health.

Learning which foods are best for your unique needs–and understanding which ones may harm your health–can empower you to find balance and achieve a healthier, more vibrant lifestyle. Nutrition, humanity's earliest form of medicine, is not just a pathway to wellness but also a connection to our roots, equipping us for a future filled with possibilities.

I invite you to explore how nutrition can become your strongest ally in easing ailments, building resilience, and fostering happiness. Are you ready to embrace this journey of discovery and transformation? Your well-being is within your control, and every meal is a chance to create a life of greater health and vitality.

Start today: Nourish your body, refresh your mind, and live fully.

Cooking Techniques

Healthy cooking is essential for everyone, especially after the age of 40. Below are various cooking techniques along with their related health benefits and potential risks.

Healthier Ways of Cooking

‣ **Steaming**: Steaming is an excellent method for preserving nutrients, as it does not require the use of additional fats. It helps keep food tender and juicy while being a gentle cooking technique that does not contribute to the formation of harmful compounds.

‣ **Oven roasting**: Oven roasting is a healthy option that does not require added oils. Foods like vegetables, fish, and chicken can be roasted in the oven to create nutritious and flavorful meals.

▸ **Light sautéing**: This method involves quickly cooking food over high heat with a small amount of healthy oil, such as olive or coconut oil. Light sautéing helps maintain the food's texture and nutrients while cooking it efficiently.

▸ **Boiling**: Boiling is a healthy cooking method, particularly for vegetables. It preserves nutrients and creates a tender texture. However, it is crucial to avoid overcooking to minimize nutrient loss.

▸ **Baking**: Baking is an excellent way to prepare food without the need for added oils. Foods like fish, poultry, vegetables, and whole grains can be baked for healthy and flavorful dishes.

Less Healthy Ways of Cooking

▸ **Frying**: Frying involves submerging food in hot oil, which significantly increases its saturated fat and calorie content. Additionally, frying at high temperatures can produce harmful compounds that pose health risks.

▸ **Breading and battering**: Coating food in breading or batter increases its calorie and fat content. These coatings can absorb more oil during cooking, resulting in a less nutritious meal.

▸ **Creamy sauces and dressings**: Cream-based sauces and dressings often contain high levels of saturated fat and excess calories. These can contribute to inflammation and exacerbate pain.

▸ **Grilling at high temperatures**: Cooking food on the grill at high heat can generate harmful compounds, such as polycyclic aromatic hydrocarbons (PAHs) and heterocyclic amines (HCAs), which have been associated with an increased cancer risk. Additionally, grilled meats can produce inflammatory substances.

Remember, the way you cook food significantly impacts its nutritional value and its overall effects on your health. Choosing healthy cooking methods ensures you maximize the benefits of your meals while reducing potential negative effects.

Nutrition, Foods, and SIBO

SIBO, or small intestinal bacterial overgrowth, is a digestive condition where bacteria that typically reside in the colon multiply excessively and migrate into the small intestine, where their presence in large numbers can cause problems. This imbalance often disrupts digestion and affects nutrient absorption, leading to uncomfortable symptoms like bloating, gas, diarrhea, or constipation–all of which can take a toll on your daily life and overall well-being.

The good news? Diet plays a powerful role in managing SIBO. Some foods can worsen symptoms, while others provide relief and help restore balance. Since everyone's body reacts differently, learning to recognize your personal food triggers is key. With the right approach, you can reduce discomfort, regain control, and feel better every day.

Take fermentable carbohydrates, for example–what's often referred to as FODMAPs (fermentable oligosaccharides, disaccharides, monosaccharides, and polyols). These include certain fruits like apples, pears, and cherries; vegetables such as onions, garlic, and cauliflower; as well as dairy, legumes, and artificial sweeteners. While these foods are healthy for many, they ferment in the small intestine for those with SIBO, resulting in gas, bloating, and discomfort. Avoiding or limiting high-FODMAP foods can be transformative in managing symptoms.

In addition, diets high in refined sugars and simple carbohydrates–such as processed foods, white bread, and sugary treats–can encourage bacterial overgrowth. Opting for a low-FODMAP diet and integrating soluble fiber-rich foods like oatmeal, carrots, and berries into your meals can help by soothing the gut, promoting better motility, and fostering balance in your digestive system.

But it's not just about what you eat–it's also about how. Eating slowly, savoring moderate portions, and chewing food thoroughly are small but impactful steps. These habits prevent food buildup in the digestive tract, which could otherwise encourage bacterial growth and magnify symptoms.

Another critical piece of the puzzle is gastric acidity, which helps eliminate harmful bacteria before they reach the small intestine. Issues such as chronic gastritis or prolonged use of acid-reducing medications can increase your risk of SIBO. If this applies to you, tackling these underlying factors with the help of a healthcare provider is essential for long-term relief.

SIBO not only affects digestion but can also lead to deficiencies in crucial nutrients, including fat-soluble vitamins (A, D, E, and K), B vitamins, iron, calcium, and zinc. Monitoring these levels and, if necessary, incorporating medical-grade supplements is vital for maintaining balance and good health.

Beyond diet, there are certain foods and supplements with natural antibacterial and anti-inflammatory benefits that may help. Ingredients like oregano oil, turmeric, ginger, and processed garlic are known to support gut health. Preparing meals with gentle methods like steaming, boiling, or baking can further reduce intestinal irritation, while frying is best avoided.

Stress management is another powerful tool for controlling SIBO. Chronic stress has a profound impact on digestion, slowing motility and weakening the immune system—factors that make bacterial overgrowth more likely. Practices such as mindfulness, meditation, yoga, or even taking moments to breathe deeply can help restore harmony between your mind and gut.

Finally, staying hydrated and following a consistent meal schedule are simple yet impactful practices. Drinking plenty of water supports digestion and eases intestinal transit, while evenly spacing your meals throughout the day helps avoid putting undue strain on your digestive system.

By adopting mindful eating habits, managing stress, and embracing a few positive lifestyle changes, you can take charge of your SIBO journey. These steps won't just ease your symptoms–they'll help you feel empowered, healthier, and more in tune with your body. Remember, every small effort can make a big difference in your quality of life.

Foods and Drinks That Commonly Cause Problems

Living with SIBO can be challenging, especially when certain foods and drinks tend to intensify symptoms. This often happens because some foods ferment quickly in the small intestine, fueling bacterial overgrowth and triggering discomfort such as bloating, gas, or abdominal pain. Among the most common culprits are fermentable carbohydrates, widely recognized as FODMAPs (fermentable oligosaccharides, disaccharides, monosaccharides, and polyols).

Dairy products also deserve attention, as they can be difficult to digest for individuals with lactose intolerance. Additionally, foods high in insoluble fiber are often problematic, as they may irritate an already sensitive digestive system. Understanding these potential triggers is the first step toward minimizing symptoms and feeling better every day.

List of trigger foods and approximate percentages:

▸ **FODMAPs**: Foods abundant in FODMAPs include onions, garlic, wheat, select vegetables (such as broccoli, cauliflower, asparagus, and mushrooms), fruits (such as apples, pears, and watermelon), and legumes (like lentils, chickpeas, and beans). Due to their fermentable nature in the small intestine, these items typically induce discomfort in roughly 75% of individuals with SIBO.

▸ **Dairy**: Dairy products, particularly those with lactose content, such as milk, cheese, and yogurt, can trigger symptoms in about 60% of people with SIBO. Lactose intolerance is prevalent among individuals with SIBO, as an abundance of bacteria in the small intestine can impede lactose digestion.

▸ **Foods rich in insoluble fiber**: While fiber is beneficial for digestive health, foods high in insoluble fiber, such as whole grains and certain vegetables, can exacerbate symptoms in approximately 50% of individuals with SIBO. Insoluble fiber can potentially heighten fermentation in the small intestine, resulting in gastrointestinal discomfort.

Each individual with SIBO is unique, and tolerance to certain foods can vary greatly from one person to another. Therefore, it is essential to follow a personalized process of food elimination and reintroduction to identify which specific foods trigger symptoms in each case. This approach not only helps to relieve discomfort but also enables the development of a more customized and sustainable long-term diet.

Below is a list of foods, along with an estimated percentage of individuals with SIBO who commonly experience discomfort when consuming them:

1. Dairy: 65%
2. Fructose: 60%
3. Chickpeas: 55%
4. Gluten: 50%
5. Beans: 50%
6. Lentils: 50%
7. Onions: 50%
8. Garlic: 50%
9. Broccoli: 45%
10. Cauliflower: 45%
11. Fiber-rich foods: 45%
12. Artificial sweeteners: 45%
13. Soft drinks: 40%
14. Mushrooms: 40%
15. Starch-rich foods: 40%
16. Rice, bread, pasta, and potatoes: approximately 30-35%

These percentages are for guidance only and may vary from one person to another, as each body responds differently. It is crucial to pay close attention to your body's reactions. Maintaining a food journal can help you identify patterns, determine which foods work well for you, and pinpoint those that may be exacerbating your symptoms. This practice will allow you to tailor your diet to your specific needs with greater confidence and precision.

Beneficial Foods for SIBO

Selecting the right foods is crucial for managing symptoms and improving quality of life. It's not only about avoiding foods that can exacerbate the condition but also about including options that offer nutritional value and are well tolerated. These foods support balanced digestion while minimizing the risk of bacterial overgrowth in the small intestine.

▸ **Lean proteins**: Chicken, turkey, fish, eggs, and tofu are excellent sources of essential nutrients and are less likely to trigger SIBO symptoms than high-fat proteins.

▸ **Low FODMAP vegetables**: Certain vegetables are less likely to trigger symptoms due to their low FODMAP content. Examples include carrots, zucchini, cucumbers, spinach, eggplants, and peppers. Green leafy vegetables are typically well tolerated.

▸ **Healthy fats**: Olive oil, coconut oil, nuts, and seeds offer essential nutrients and are less likely to aggravate SIBO symptoms than saturated fats.

▸ **Moderate starch intake**: While starchy foods may exacerbate symptoms for some individuals, others can tolerate moderate amounts of well-cooked starches like white rice and skinless potatoes.

▸ **Probiotics and fermented foods**: Natural probiotics found in lactose-free yogurt, kefir, sauerkraut, and kimchi are often beneficial for individuals with SIBO, aiding in restoring a healthy bacterial balance in the gut.

▸ **Bone broth**: Homemade bone broth can be easily digested and provides nutrients beneficial for gastrointestinal health.

In addition to the foods mentioned above, there are others

that may benefit individuals with SIBO:

▸ **Fish and shellfish:** These lean protein sources also contain omega-3 fatty acids, which are known for their anti-inflammatory properties and potential benefits for gut health.

▸ **Coconut oil:** This oil contains medium-chain fatty acids that are readily digestible and can serve as an alternative energy source for intestinal cells.

▸ **Flax and chia seeds:** These are rich in soluble fiber and omega-3 fatty acids, which can benefit gut health. However, it is advisable to introduce them gradually, as they may cause discomfort in some individuals with SIBO.

▸ **Lean beef:** While beef may pose digestion challenges for some individuals with SIBO, lean meat can serve as an additional protein source rich in essential nutrients.

▸ **Low FODMAP fruits:** Certain fruits, such as ripe bananas, berries, oranges, and grapes, are less likely to trigger SIBO symptoms due to their low FODMAP content.

▸ **Pumpkin and winter squash** are low in FODMAPs and can be well-tolerated additions to the diet of individuals with SIBO.

▸ **Herbal teas:** Certain herbal teas, such as chamomile, ginger, and peppermint, can help relieve digestive symptoms and provide comfort.

▸ **Olive oil:** Raw, first cold-pressed extra virgin olive oil is a source of monounsaturated fatty acids with antiinflammatory properties that benefit intestinal health.

▸ **Homemade broths and soups:** These provide easily digestible nutrients and help maintain hydration, particularly during episodes of digestive distress.

▸ **Lactose-free milk and milk alternatives:** For those with limited lactose tolerance, options like lactose-free milk, almond milk, coconut milk, and other alternatives may be well-tolerated.

▸ **Eggs:** An excellent protein and nutrient source that is often well-tolerated by many individuals with SIBO.

▸ **Aloe vera juice:** Known for its soothing properties on the gastrointestinal tract and ability to provide relief.

▸ **Foods rich in soluble fiber:** Soluble fiber-rich foods, such as oats and psyllium, can regulate intestinal transit and promote digestive health.

It is important to remember that everyone responds to food differently, making it vital to understand how your body reacts. Keeping a food and symptom journal can be an invaluable tool for recognizing patterns, identifying the foods you tolerate well, and pinpointing those that may cause discomfort.

When incorporating new foods into your diet, take a slow and intentional approach. This gradual method allows you to accurately assess your tolerance, identify potential triggers, and safely tailor your diet to meet your specific needs.

Mint: Digestive Ally or Hidden Enemy?

Mint and its derivatives, such as peppermint oil, have long been used to treat various digestive issues, including irritable bowel syndrome (IBS) and indigestion. For some individuals, mint can help ease symptoms like stomach discomfort, nausea, and abdominal pain.

However, for others, mint can aggravate digestive problems. This is because it contains menthol, which has the potential to relax the lower esophageal sphincter, allowing stomach acid to flow back into the esophagus, thereby worsening acid reflux. Additionally, menthol may trigger symptoms such as heartburn, burning sensations, or general digestive discomfort in certain individuals.

In the specific case of people with small intestinal bacterial overgrowth, mint is often listed as a food to avoid. The menthol in mint can relax the muscles of the digestive tract, potentially exacerbating symptoms linked to bacterial overgrowth in the small intestine.

Understanding how your body reacts to mint is essential for determining whether it is a digestive ally or a hidden foe.

Beneficial Beverages for SIBO

If you're managing SIBO, selecting the right beverages can play a key role in alleviating your symptoms and promoting better gut health. Below is a list of options that may support your dietary plan and contribute to your overall well-being:

▸ **Water**: Maintaining proper hydration is vital for digestive health. Pure water is essential for promoting adequate bowel function, cellular hydration, and the elimination of toxins.

▸ **Herbal teas**: Chamomile, peppermint, ginger, fennel, and licorice herbal teas are often effective in relieving SIBO symptoms. Chamomile and peppermint possess soothing properties for the digestive tract, ginger aids in alleviating nausea, and fennel and licorice are recognized for their carminative properties, which help reduce bloating and abdominal discomfort.

▸ **Green tea**: Rich in antioxidants and anti-inflammatory compounds, green tea can benefit intestinal health. However, individuals with digestive sensitivities may find green tea irritating, so it is crucial to monitor individual responses.

▸ **Kombucha**: This fermented tea-based beverage frequently contains probiotics that promote gut health. However, its sugar and gas content may cause digestive discomfort for some people with SIBO, necessitating cautious consumption.

▸ **Bone broth**: Homemade bone broth is a nutrient-rich source containing minerals, collagen, and amino acids that support gut health. Additionally, bone broth aids in maintaining hydration and alleviating gastrointestinal symptoms.

‣ **Almond milk and coconut milk**: These dairy alternatives may be well-tolerated by individuals with SIBO who are lactose intolerant or have dairy sensitivities.

‣ **Aloe vera juice**: Known for its soothing properties on the digestive tract, aloe vera juice can offer relief. However, it must be diluted and consumed in moderation, as excessive intake may have a laxative effect on some individuals.

‣ **Coconut water**: A beneficial source of electrolytes, coconut water aids in hydration, which is particularly important for individuals with SIBO who experience diarrhea or fluid loss.

‣ **Ginger water**: Steeping fresh ginger slices in water provides anti-inflammatory and carminative properties that help alleviate swelling and discomfort.

‣ **Turmeric infusion**: Turmeric is recognized for its anti-inflammatory and antioxidant properties, which support gut health. It can be combined with black pepper and ginger in an infusion to enhance the bioavailability of its active components.

‣ **Hibiscus infusion**: Rich in antioxidants and compounds with anti-inflammatory properties, hibiscus infusion supports digestive health.

‣ **Carrot and ginger juice**: This juice combines fresh carrots with a touch of ginger, offering beneficial nutrients and anti-inflammatory compounds that promote gut health.

‣ **Celery juice**: Fresh celery juice is advantageous for individuals with SIBO, as it contains nutrients that nurture digestive tract health.

‣ **Lemon water**: Warm lemon water possesses alkalizing properties and boosts the production of digestive enzymes, benefiting those with SIBO.

‣ **Almond milk with turmeric and cinnamon**: This

mixture provides anti-inflammatory nutrients that support gut health, assuming the individual tolerates it well.

‣ **Water kefir**: A fermented beverage rich in probiotics, water kefir promotes gut health. Nonetheless, some individuals with SIBO may find that fermented drinks exacerbate their symptoms, emphasizing the need to monitor individual responses.

‣ **Cucumber and mint juice**: This refreshing blend may offer benefits to specific individuals with SIBO due to its high water content and the soothing properties of mint.

‣ **Coconut milk with turmeric and ginger**: This beverage supplies anti-inflammatory nutrients that support gut health.

‣ **Basil infusion**: Basil is renowned for its anti-inflammatory properties.

‣ **Dandelion infusion**: Possessing cleansing and digestive stimulant properties, dandelion infusion is advantageous for intestinal health.

‣ **Spinach and ginger juice**: This juice combines fresh spinach and ginger and provides nutrients and anti-inflammatory compounds that promote digestive tract health.

In the chapter "Juices and Smoothies," you'll find a carefully curated selection of options designed for individuals with SIBO.

Keep in mind that tolerance to these beverages can vary from person to person. While some may promote better gut health and help you feel your best, others might cause discomfort. It's essential to listen to your body, observe how you feel after consuming them, and adjust your diet accordingly to suit your individual needs.

Harmful Beverages

For people with SIBO, certain beverages may exacerbate symptoms and impede recovery. These often include the following:

‣ **High-sugar drinks:** Simple sugars are known to fuel bacteria in the gut. Beverages like soft drinks, commercial juices, energy drinks, and some sports drinks contain high levels of added sugars, which can worsen bacterial overgrowth in the small intestine. Consumption of these drinks increases bacterial fermentation and exacerbates SIBO symptoms.

‣ **Alcoholic beverages:** Alcohol consumption is often detrimental for individuals with SIBO. Alcohol can potentially irritate the intestinal mucosa and disrupt the balance of intestinal bacteria. Additionally, alcohol consumption frequently weakens the immune system, further hindering the body's ability to regulate bacterial overgrowth in the small intestine.

‣ **Caffeinated beverages:** Coffee and other caffeinated beverages can prompt acid production in the stomach, impacting intestinal motility and worsening SIBO symptoms. Furthermore, caffeine can lead to dehydration, which can affect the overall health of the gastrointestinal tract.

‣ **Dairy drinks:** Dairy beverages like milk and certain types of milkshakes can pose issues for individuals with SIBO, particularly those who are lactose intolerant. Undigested lactose can ferment in the small intestine, exacerbating symptoms.

‣ **Carbonated beverages:** Carbonated beverages, including artificially sweetened ones, can exacerbate bloating and abdominal discomfort. The effervescent bubbles in these drinks can intensify existing symptoms.

In addition to avoiding the beverages mentioned, you may benefit from **reducing or eliminating those that contain artificial sweeteners such as sorbitol, mannitol, and**

xylitol. These sweeteners often ferment in the gut, potentially worsening your symptoms and delaying your recovery.

Keep in mind that everyone is unique, and what works for one person might not work for you. You may tolerate some of these beverages in small amounts, or it might be best to avoid them entirely to support your gut health. Paying close attention to your body's signals will be key to finding the balance that works best for you.

SIBO Support: Easy and Tasty Recipes

Explore a collection of simple, flavorful recipes specially crafted for those who want to nurture their digestive health while savoring delicious, SIBO-friendly meals!

Breakfast Options

1. Yoghurt and fruit bowl:

Ingredients: 1 cup lactose-free yogurt or plant-based milk, 1/2 cup mixed berries, 1 tablespoon chia seeds, 1 tablespoon chopped walnuts.

Preparation: Place the yogurt in a bowl and add the berries, chia seeds, and walnuts. Mix well, then enjoy.

2. Omelette with egg whites and spinach:

Ingredients: 4 egg whites, a handful of fresh spinach, salt and pepper to taste.

Preparation: Beat the egg whites in a bowl and add the spinach. Add salt and pepper to taste. Cook the omelet in a non-stick frying pan until firm. Serve warm.

3. Banana and oatmeal pancakes:

Ingredients: 1 ripe banana, 1/2 cup gluten-free oat flour, 2 eggs, 1 teaspoon ground cinnamon, 1 teaspoon coconut oil.

Preparation: Mash the banana in a bowl and add the oat flour, eggs, and cinnamon. Mix well until you obtain a homogeneous dough. Heat the coconut oil in a nonstick frying pan and pour in small portions of the batter to make the pancakes. Cook on both sides until golden brown. Serve with fresh fruit.

4. Protein and fruit shake:

Ingredients: 1 cup unsweetened almond milk, 1 scoop protein powder without dairy or added sugars, 1/2 cup frozen mixed berries, and 1 tablespoon almond butter.

Preparation: Place all ingredients in a blender and blend until smooth. Serve cold.

5. Quinoa bowl with fruit:

Ingredients: 1/2 cup cooked quinoa, 1/2 cup unsweetened almond milk, 1 teaspoon ground cinnamon, 1 tablespoon chia seeds, and 1/4 cup chopped fresh fruit (such as strawberries, bananas, or blueberries).

Preparation: In a bowl, combine the cooked quinoa, almond milk, cinnamon and chia seeds. Mix well and let stand for 10 minutes to allow the chia seeds to hydrate. Then top with fresh fruit and enjoy.

6. Spinach and pineapple smoothie:

Ingredients: 1 cup fresh spinach, 1 cup fresh pineapple, 1/2 banana, 1 cup unsweetened coconut milk.

Preparation: Combine all ingredients in a blender and blend until smooth. To make it more refreshing, add ice. Serve chilled.

7. Spinach and mushroom omelette:

Ingredients: 3 eggs, a handful of fresh spinach, 4-5 mushrooms, salt and pepper to taste.

Preparation: In a non-stick pan, sauté the spinach and mushrooms until tender. In a bowl, beat the eggs and add salt and pepper to taste. Pour the beaten eggs over the spinach and mushrooms in the skillet. Cook over medium-low heat until the egg is firm. Serve hot.

8. Whey protein shake and almond butter:

Ingredients: 1 cup unsweetened almond milk, 1 scoop whey protein with no dairy or added sugars, 1 scoop almond butter, 1/2 frozen banana.

Preparation: Combine all ingredients in a blender and blend until smooth. To make it more refreshing, add ice. Serve chilled.

Lunch Creations

1. Chicken and avocado salad:
Ingredients: Grilled chicken breast in chunks, lettuce leaves, sliced avocado, cherry tomato, sliced cucumber, olive oil, lemon juice, salt and pepper to taste.

Preparation: In a large bowl, mix lettuce leaves, grilled chicken, avocado, cherry tomato and cucumber. Dress with olive oil, lemon juice, salt, and pepper to taste. Mix well and serve.

2. Baked salmon with roasted vegetables:
Ingredients: Salmon fillet, broccoli, carrots, courgette, olive oil, salt, and spices to taste.

Preparation: Preheat the oven to 200°C. Place the salmon fillet and the diced vegetables in an ovenproof dish. Drizzle with olive oil and season with salt and spices to taste. Bake for approximately 20-25 minutes until the salmon is cooked and the vegetables are tender.

3. Quinoa and vegetable salad:
Ingredients: Cooked quinoa, diced cucumber, diced tomato, diced red pepper, pitted olives, chopped mint leaves, lemon juice, olive oil, salt and pepper to taste.

Preparation: Combine cooked quinoa, cucumber, tomato, red pepper, olives, and mint in a large bowl. Dress with lemon juice, olive oil, salt, and pepper to taste. Mix well and serve.

4. Grilled chicken breasts with cauliflower puree:
Ingredients: Chicken breasts, cauliflower chunks, fat-free chicken stock, olive oil, salt and spices.

Preparation: In a nonstick frying pan, cook the grilled chicken breasts with olive oil, salt, and spices to taste. Meanwhile, boil the cauliflower in the chicken stock until tender. Drain the liquid and mash the cauliflower with a fork or food processor to a puree-like texture. Serve the chicken breasts with the cauliflower puree.

5. Pumpkin and ginger soup:
Ingredients: 1 small pumpkin, peeled and cut into chunks, 1

tablespoon grated fresh ginger, 1 chopped onion, 2 chopped garlic cloves, fat-free chicken stock, salt, and pepper to taste.

Preparation: In a large pot, sauté the onion and garlic until tender. Add the pumpkin and grated ginger, and cook for a few more minutes. Add enough chicken stock to cover the ingredients and bring to a boil. Reduce the heat and simmer until the pumpkin is tender. Remove from the heat and puree the soup with an immersion blender or a food processor until smooth. Add salt and pepper to taste. Serve hot.

6. Salmon and avocado salad:

Ingredients: Shredded grilled salmon fillet, spinach leaves, sliced avocado, diced tomato, sliced cucumber, olive oil, lemon juice, salt, and pepper to taste.

Preparation: Place the spinach leaves on a large plate. Add the shredded salmon, avocado, tomato, and cucumber. Dress with olive oil, lemon juice, salt, and pepper to taste. Mix well and serve.

7. Curried chicken with cauliflower and spinach:

Ingredients: Diced chicken breast, cauliflower in small pieces, fresh spinach, unsweetened coconut milk, red curry paste, coconut oil, salt and spices to taste.

Preparation: Heat the coconut oil over medium-high heat in a large skillet and add the chicken. Cook until golden brown on all sides. Add the cauliflower and red curry paste and cook for a few more minutes. Then add the coconut milk and spinach. Simmer until the cauliflower is tender and the spinach has wilted, and season with salt and spices to taste. Serve hot.

8. Quinoa salad with shrimp:

Ingredients: Cooked quinoa, cooked and peeled shrimp, diced cucumber, cherry tomatoes, pitted olives, chopped parsley leaves, lemon juice, olive oil, salt, and pepper to taste.

Preparation: Combine cooked quinoa, shrimp, cucumber, tomato, olives, and parsley in a large bowl. Dress with lemon juice, olive oil, salt, and pepper to taste. Mix well and serve.

9. Grilled chicken with grilled vegetables:

Ingredients: Grilled chicken breast, sliced courgette, sliced aubergine, diced peppers, olive oil, salt and spices to taste.

Preparation: Grill the chicken breast on a grill or grill pan until cooked through. Meanwhile, cook the courgette, aubergine, and peppers in a nonstick frying pan with olive oil, salt, and spices to taste until tender and lightly browned. Serve the chicken along with the grilled vegetables.

10. Lettuce tacos with ground beef:

Ingredients: Lean ground beef, large lettuce leaves, chopped onion, garlic, cumin, paprika, salt and spices to taste.

Preparation: In a nonstick pan, cook the ground beef with the onion and garlic until cooked through. Add cumin, paprika, salt, and spices to taste. Wash and dry the lettuce leaves and use them as "tortillas" to make tacos. Fill each lettuce leaf with ground beef and add your favorite toppings, such as tomato, avocado, cilantro, etc.

11. Baked fish with herb sauce:

Ingredients: Fish fillet (such as salmon, sole, or sea bass), lemon juice, olive oil, chopped parsley, basil, mint, salt, and pepper to taste.

Preparation: Preheat the oven to 200°C. Place the fish fillet on a baking tray and sprinkle it with lemon juice, olive oil, salt, and pepper to taste. Mix the chopped parsley, basil, and mint leaves in a bowl. Sprinkle the herb mixture over the fish. Bake for approximately 15-20 minutes, or until the fish is cooked through and flakes easily with a fork.

12. Chickpea and vegetable salad:

Ingredients: Cooked chickpeas, diced cucumber, diced tomato, diced green pepper, thinly sliced red onion, chopped parsley leaves, lemon juice, olive oil, salt and pepper to taste.

Preparation: Combine cooked chickpeas, cucumber, tomato, green pepper, red onion, and parsley in a large bowl. Add lemon juice, olive oil, salt, and pepper to taste. Mix well and serve.

13. Lettuce rolls with chicken and vegetables:

Ingredients: Cooked shredded chicken breast, large lettuce leaves, shredded carrot, shredded cabbage, cucumber strips, low-sodium soy sauce, sesame oil, rice vinegar, salt, and spices to taste.

Preparation: In a bowl, mix the shredded chicken with the shredded carrot, cabbage, and cucumber. Mix the soy sauce, sesame oil, rice vinegar, salt, and spices in another bowl to taste and make the dressing. Place a portion of the chicken and vegetable mixture on a lettuce leaf and drizzle with the dressing. Roll up the lettuce leaf and secure it with chopsticks. Serve cold.

14. Peppers stuffed with pork and rice:

Ingredients: Peppers (red, yellow, or green), ground pork, cooked white rice, chopped onion, chopped garlic, diced tomato, fat-free chicken stock, salt, and spices to taste.

Preparation: Preheat the oven to 180°C. Cut the tops off the peppers and remove the seeds and membranes. In a frying pan, cook the ground pork with the onion and garlic until cooked through. Add the tomato and cook for a few more minutes. Add the cooked rice and chicken stock, and season with salt and spices to taste. Stuff the peppers with the meat and rice mixture. Place on a baking sheet and bake for approximately 30-40 minutes or until the peppers are tender.

15. Tuna and chickpea salad:

Ingredients: Canned tuna in water, cooked chickpeas, diced cucumber, diced tomato, thinly sliced red onion, chopped parsley leaves, lemon juice, olive oil, salt and pepper to taste.

Preparation: In a large bowl, combine shredded tuna, cooked chickpeas, cucumber, tomato, red onion, and parsley. Add lemon juice, olive oil, salt, and pepper to taste. Mix well and serve.

16. Chicken curry with sautéed vegetables:

Ingredients: Diced chicken breast, mixed vegetables (such as carrots, broccoli, and peppers), unsweetened coconut milk, yellow curry paste, coconut oil, salt, and spices to taste.

Preparation: Heat the coconut oil in a large skillet and add the chicken. Cook until golden brown on all sides. Add the vegetable mixture and cook for a few more minutes. Then, add the coconut milk and yellow curry paste. Simmer until the vegetables are tender, and season with salt and spices to taste. Serve hot.

17. Salmon and avocado salad:

Ingredients: Cooked and flaked salmon fillet, diced avocado, cucumber, tomato, spinach leaves, lemon juice, olive oil, salt, and pepper to taste.

Preparation: Combine the flaked salmon, avocado, cucumber, tomato, and spinach leaves in a large bowl. Dress with lemon juice, olive oil, salt, and pepper to taste. Mix well and serve.

18. Egg white omelette with vegetables:

Ingredients: Egg whites, chopped spinach, sliced mushrooms, chopped onion, diced red pepper, olive oil, salt and spices to taste.

Preparation: Heat a little olive oil in a nonstick frying pan over medium heat. Add the onion and red pepper and cook until tender. Add the spinach and mushrooms and cook for a few more minutes. Whisk the egg whites with salt and spices in another bowl to taste. Pour the egg whites over the vegetables in the pan and cook until firm on one side. Flip the omelet and cook on the other side until cooked through. Serve warm.

19. Chicken and vegetable soup:

Ingredients: Cooked and shredded chicken breast, fat-free chicken broth, sliced carrot, chopped celery, chopped onion, chopped garlic, chopped parsley leaves, olive oil, salt and spices to taste.

Preparation: Heat a little olive oil over medium heat in a large pot. Add the onion, garlic, celery, and carrot, and cook until tender. Add the chicken stock and bring to the boil. Reduce the heat and add the shredded chicken breast. Simmer for a few minutes to allow the flavors to blend, and season it with salt and spices to taste. Serve hot.

20. Quinoa salad with roasted vegetables:

Ingredients: Cooked quinoa, roasted peppers in strips, diced roasted courgette, aubergine, tomato, rocket leaves, lemon juice, olive oil, salt and pepper to taste.

Preparation: Combine cooked quinoa, roasted peppers, roasted courgette, aubergine, tomato, and arugula leaves in a large bowl. Dress with lemon juice, olive oil, salt, and pepper to taste. Mix well and serve.

Snacks

1. Turkey and cucumber rolls:

Ingredients: 4-6 slices of turkey, 1 cucumber, 1/4 avocado.
Preparation: Cut the cucumber into long, thin strips. Spread each slice of turkey with a small amount of avocado. Then, wrap the cucumber strips with the turkey slices. Enjoy these fresh and tasty rolls.

2. Carrot sticks with chickpea hummus:

Ingredients: 2 carrots, 1/2 cup cooked chickpeas, 1 tablespoon tahini, 1 tablespoon olive oil, half a lemon juice, salt, and spices to taste.
Preparation: Peel the carrots and cut them into sticks. For the hummus, combine the chickpeas, tahini, olive oil, lemon juice, salt, and spices in a food processor and blend until smooth. Serve the carrot sticks with the hummus.

3. Baked kale chips:

Ingredients: Kale leaves, olive oil, salt, and spices to taste.
Preparation: Preheat the oven to 150°C. Wash and dry the kale leaves and remove the stems. In a bowl, add a little olive oil, salt, and spices to taste. Massage the kale leaves with this mixture until well coated. Place the leaves on a baking sheet and bake for 10-15 minutes or until crisp. Allow them to cool before enjoying.

4. Mini vegetable frittatas:

Ingredients: 4 eggs, 1 cup chopped vegetables (such as spinach, peppers, mushrooms), salt, and spices to taste.
Preparation: Preheat the oven to 180°C. Beat the eggs in a bowl and add the chopped vegetables, salt, and spices to taste. Pour the mixture into greased or baking paper-lined muffin tins. Bake for 15-20 minutes or until the frittatas are cooked. Let them cool before eating.

5. Cucumber and salmon rolls:

Ingredients: 1 cucumber, 100 g smoked salmon, 1 tablespoon lactose-free cream cheese, lemon juice, chopped fresh dill.
Preparation: Cut the cucumber into long, thin strips. Mix the cream cheese, lemon juice, and dill in a bowl. Spread a thin

layer of this mixture on each cucumber strip and place a slice of salmon on top. Roll up the cucumber and secure it with a toothpick. Serve cold.

6. Almond and date energy balls:

Ingredients: 1 cup almonds, 1 cup pitted dates, 2 tablespoons unsweetened cocoa powder, 1 tablespoon coconut oil.

Preparation: Blend the almonds, dates, cocoa powder, and coconut oil in a food processor until the dough is sticky. Form the dough into small balls and refrigerate for at least 1 hour before eating.

7. Homemade popcorn:

Ingredients: 1/2 cup popcorn kernels, 1 tablespoon coconut oil, salt, and spices to taste.

Preparation: Heat a large pot with a lid over medium-high heat and add the coconut oil. Add the popcorn kernels and cover the pot with the lid. Cook, stirring occasionally, until popcorn is popped. Remove from heat and season with salt and spices to taste.

8. Green detox smoothie:

Ingredients: 1 cup fresh spinach, 1/2 cucumber, 1/2 green apple, juice of half a lemon, 1 cup coconut water.

Preparation: Combine all ingredients in a blender and blend until smooth. To make it more refreshing, add ice. Serve chilled.

Dinner Ideas

1. Baked salmon with asparagus:
Ingredients: Salmon fillet, asparagus, olive oil, lemon juice, salt, and spices to taste.

Preparation: Preheat the oven to 180°C. Place the salmon on a baking tray and season it with salt, spices, and lemon juice to taste. Arrange the asparagus around the salmon and drizzle with olive oil. Bake for approximately 15-20 minutes, until the salmon is cooked and the asparagus is tender. Serve hot.

2. Grilled chicken with spinach and strawberry salad:
Ingredients: Chicken breast, fresh spinach, chopped walnuts, sliced strawberries, balsamic vinegar, olive oil, salt and pepper to taste.

Preparation: Season the chicken breast with salt and pepper to taste. Grill until cooked through. In a large bowl, mix spinach, strawberries and walnuts. Dress with balsamic vinegar and olive oil. Mix well and serve with grilled chicken.

3. Lettuce rolls with ground beef and vegetables:
Ingredients: Ground beef or turkey, large lettuce leaves, shredded carrot, diced courgette, chopped onion, chopped garlic, fish sauce, sesame oil, salt, and spices to taste.

Preparation: Heat a little sesame oil over medium heat in a large frying pan. Add the onion and garlic and cook until tender. Add the ground beef and cook until it is cooked through. Add the grated carrot and courgette, and cook for a few more minutes. Season with fish sauce, salt, and spices to taste. Roll up some meat and vegetable mixture on a lettuce leaf. Serve cold.

4. Chicken and avocado salad:
Ingredients: Cooked and shredded chicken breast, diced avocado, cucumber, tomato, lettuce leaves, lemon juice, olive oil, salt, and pepper to taste.

Preparation: Combine shredded chicken, avocado, cucumber, tomato, and lettuce leaves in a large bowl. Dress with lemon juice, olive oil, salt, and pepper to taste. Mix well and serve.

5. Baked fish with asparagus and cherry tomatoes:

Ingredients: Fish fillet (hake, sea bass, etc.), asparagus, cherry tomatoes, olive oil, lemon juice, salt, and spices to taste.

Preparation: Preheat the oven to 180°C. Place the fish on a baking tray and season it with salt, spices, and lemon juice to taste. Add the asparagus and cherry tomatoes around the fish and drizzle with olive oil. Bake for 15-20 minutes until the fish is cooked and the asparagus is tender. Serve hot.

6. Shrimp and avocado salad:

Ingredients: Cooked and peeled shrimp, diced avocado, cucumber, tomato, spinach leaves, lemon juice, olive oil, salt, and pepper to taste.

Preparation: Combine shrimp, avocado, cucumber, tomato, and spinach leaves in a large bowl. Dress with lemon juice, olive oil, salt, and pepper to taste. Mix well and serve.

7. Chicken curry with vegetables:

Ingredients: Diced chicken breast, sliced carrot, diced courgette, chopped onion, chopped garlic, coconut milk, red curry paste, coconut oil, salt and spices to taste.

Preparation: Heat a little coconut oil over medium heat in a large frying pan. Add the onion and garlic and cook until tender. Add the chicken and cook until cooked through. Add the carrot and courgette and cook for a few more minutes. Mix the red curry paste with the coconut milk and add to the pan. Simmer until the flavors blend and the vegetables are tender, seasoned with salt and spices to taste. Serve hot.

8. Peppers stuffed with quinoa and vegetables:

Ingredients: Peppers (red, green, or yellow), cooked quinoa, chopped onion, diced courgette, chopped mushrooms, diced tomato, olive oil, salt, and spices to taste.

Preparation: Preheat the oven to 180°C. Cut the peppers' tops off and remove the seeds. Heat a little olive oil in a large frying pan over medium heat. Add the onion, courgette, mushrooms, and tomato, and cook until tender. Add the cooked quinoa and season with salt and spices to taste. Stuff the peppers with the quinoa and vegetable mixture. Place the peppers on a baking sheet and bake for approximately 30-40 minutes or until tender. Serve hot.

9. Pumpkin and ginger soup:

Ingredients: Diced pumpkin, chopped onion, chopped garlic, grated ginger, fat-free chicken stock, olive oil, salt, and spices to taste.

Preparation: Heat a little olive oil over medium heat in a large pot. Add the onion, garlic and ginger, and cook until tender. Add the pumpkin and sauté for a few minutes. Add the chicken stock, salt, and spices to taste. Cook over medium-low heat until the pumpkin is tender and can be easily mashed. Remove from heat and puree the soup with a blender or food processor until smooth. Reheat the soup before serving.

10. Lettuce tacos with beef and guacamole:

Ingredients: Lean ground beef, lettuce leaves, diced tomato, chopped onion, chopped coriander, lime juice, olive oil, salt and spices to taste.

Preparation: Heat a little olive oil in a large frying pan over medium heat. Add the onion and cook until tender. Add the ground beef and cook until it is cooked through and seasoned with salt and spices to taste. Wash and dry the lettuce leaves. Stuff each leaf with the meat and add tomato, onion, and chopped coriander. Prepare guacamole by mixing diced avocado with lime juice, salt, and spices. Serve the lettuce tacos with guacamole.

11. Baked turkey with cauliflower puree:

Ingredients: Turkey breast, cauliflower florets, fat-free chicken stock, olive oil, salt, and spices to taste.

Preparation: Preheat the oven to 180°C. Place the turkey breast on a baking tray and season with salt and spices to taste. Bake until the turkey is cooked through and nice and juicy. Meanwhile, cook the cauliflower in chicken stock until tender. Drain the cauliflower and puree it with a blender or food processor to achieve a smooth consistency. Add olive oil, salt, and spices to taste. Serve the baked turkey with the cauliflower puree.

12. Smoked salmon and rocket salad:

Ingredients: Smoked salmon chunks, rocket, sliced cucumber, diced tomato, black olives, lemon juice, olive oil, salt and pepper to taste.

Preparation: In a large bowl, mix the rocket, cucumber, tomato, and olives. Add the smoked salmon pieces. Dress with lemon juice, olive oil, salt, and pepper to taste. Mix well and serve.

13. Grilled chicken with asparagus and feta cheese:

Ingredients: Chicken breast, asparagus, crumbled feta cheese, olive oil, lemon juice, salt and spices.

Preparation: Season the chicken breast with salt, spices, and lemon juice to taste. Grill the chicken until cooked through. Meanwhile, sauté the asparagus in olive oil in a separate pan until tender. Serve the chicken with the asparagus and sprinkle feta cheese on top.

14. Salmon and avocado salad:

Ingredients: Salmon fillet, diced avocado, sliced cucumber, diced tomato, spinach leaves, lemon juice, olive oil, salt and pepper to taste.

Preparation: Grill or bake the salmon until cooked through. Shred it into smaller pieces. Mix the salmon, avocado, cucumber, tomato, and spinach leaves in a large bowl. Dress with lemon juice, olive oil, salt, and pepper to taste. Mix well and serve.

15. Peppers stuffed with ground beef and vegetables:

Ingredients: Peppers (red, green, or yellow), lean ground beef, chopped onion, diced courgette, chopped mushrooms, tomato, olive oil, salt, and spices.

Preparation: Preheat the oven to 180°C. Cut the tops off the peppers and remove the seeds. Heat a little olive oil over medium heat in a large frying pan. Add the onion, courgette, mushrooms, and tomato, and cook until tender. Add the ground beef and cook until it is cooked through. Season with salt and spices to taste. Stuff the peppers with the ground beef and vegetable mixture. Place the peppers on a baking sheet and bake for approximately 30-40 minutes or until tender. Serve hot.

16. Chicken and vegetable soup:

Ingredients: Chicken breast, sliced carrot, diced courgette, fat-free chicken stock, chopped onion, chopped garlic, olive oil, salt and spices to taste.

Preparation: Heat a little olive oil over medium heat in a large pot. Add the onion and garlic and cook until tender. Add the chicken breast and cook until cooked through. Remove the chicken breast from the pan and shred it into smaller pieces. Return the shredded chicken to the pot along with the carrots, courgette, and chicken stock. Cook over medium-low heat until the vegetables are tender. Season with salt and spices to taste. Serve hot.

17. Baked fish with asparagus and lemon:

Ingredients: Fish fillet (such as hake or sole), asparagus, lemon slices, olive oil, salt, and spices to taste.

Preparation: Preheat the oven to 180°C. Place the fish fillet on a baking tray and season with salt, spices, and olive oil. Arrange the asparagus around the fish and add the lemon slices. Bake for approximately 15-20 minutes until the fish is cooked through and the asparagus is tender. Serve hot.

18. Chicken salad with avocado and spinach:

Ingredients: Chicken breast, diced avocado, spinach leaves, diced tomato, chopped walnuts, lemon juice, olive oil, salt and pepper to taste.

Preparation: Grill or bake the chicken breast until cooked through. Shred into smaller pieces. Mix the shredded chicken, avocado, spinach leaves, tomato, and walnuts in a large bowl. Dress with lemon juice, olive oil, salt, and pepper to taste. Mix well and serve.

19. Turkey casserole with vegetables:

Ingredients: Diced turkey breast, diced butternut squash, sliced carrot, spinach, fat-free chicken stock, chopped onion, chopped garlic, olive oil, salt and spices to taste.

Preparation: Heat a little olive oil in a large pot over medium heat. Add the onion and garlic and cook until tender. Add the turkey breast and cook until cooked through. Add the pumpkin, carrot, and chicken stock and cook over medium-low heat until the vegetables are tender. Add the spinach and cook for a few more minutes until wilted and seasoned with salt and spices to taste. Serve hot.

20. Spinach and feta omelette:

Ingredients: Eggs, chopped spinach, crumbled feta cheese, chopped onion, olive oil, salt and spices to taste.

Preparation: Heat olive oil in a nonstick frying pan over medium heat. Add the onion and cook until tender. Add the spinach and cook until wilted. In a separate bowl, beat the eggs with salt and spices to taste. Pour the egg mixture over the spinach and sprinkle the feta cheese. Cook the omelet over medium-low heat until firm and golden brown on both sides. Serve warm.

Remember to adapt the recipes to your personal needs and tolerances - I hope you enjoy these delicious recipes!

JUICES AND SMOOTHIES

"Fresh juices are the elixir of life, a powerful source of nutrients" (Norman Walker)

Raw foods, often referred to as "living" foods, are an exceptional source of vitamins, minerals, fiber, trace elements, enzymes, and other vital compounds that support overall health. Incorporating these nutrient-rich foods into your daily diet not only aids in disease prevention but also alleviates symptoms of various health conditions, slows down the aging process, balances gut flora, and enhances energy levels and vitality.

While salads, whole fruits, and nuts are excellent raw food options, one of the easiest and most convenient ways to ensure regular intake is by preparing homemade juices, smoothies, and shakes. These beverages serve as a delicious and practical alternative for individuals who may not enjoy consuming fruits and vegetables directly, making it easier to include these essential nutrients in their diet.

In today's world, where ultra-processed foods and toxins have become increasingly prevalent, the need for natural, nutrient-dense foods is more crucial than ever. Raw foods play a vital role in supporting detoxification, maintaining health, and restoring balance to the body.

Many people tend to prepare their juices and smoothies using only fruits, often overlooking the incredible health benefits vegetables and leafy greens provide. Adding these to your recipes not only increases variety but also significantly boosts their nutritional value, enhancing their antioxidant, remineralizing, toning, and alkalizing properties. These qualities help maintain the body's balance, rejuvenate cells, and promote overall well-being. Additionally, vegetables and greens lower the glycemic index, improve satiety, and maximize the health benefits of these preparations.

However, it is crucial to understand that most store-bought juices are far from healthy options. These commercial products are often loaded with excessive added sugars, artificial sweeteners, preservatives, and harmful chemical additives. Furthermore, the pasteurization processes used during production strip away essential vitamins and enzymes, rendering them nutritionally deficient. The high level of refinement also removes fiber, a vital component of whole foods. In many cases, these juices contain only minimal amounts of actual fruit, making them highly processed and lacking true nutritional value.

One major concern with many juices and smoothies is their high glycemic index, which can cause blood sugar spikes, lead to weight gain, and contribute to long-term metabolic imbalances. To truly enjoy healthy and nourishing beverages, the best approach is to prepare them at home using fresh, natural, and high-quality ingredients. Homemade juices and smoothies are packed with nutrients that provide genuine benefits for your body and overall well-being.

Incorporating fresh juices made from fruits, vegetables, and leafy greens into your daily routine is an excellent practice for maintaining a healthy and energetic body. With endless combinations to explore, you can enjoy not only flavorful and refreshing options but also targeted health benefits, such as relief from conditions like arthritis, thanks to essential nutrients that support wellness. Making this a part of your everyday life can transform your health, boost your energy, and elevate your quality of life. Try it for yourself and feel the difference!

Homemade Juices: A Natural Relief for SIBO

Homemade juices and smoothies can be a practical and nutritious solution for individuals managing SIBO. They allow you to enjoy their benefits while addressing the symptoms of this condition. By preparing them at home, you have the chance to select specific ingredients tailored to the needs of a sensitive digestive system. Here's how incorporating home-made juices into your daily routine can support your well-being if you're living with SIBO.

When you make juices and smoothies at home, you gain full control over the ingredients. This means you can avoid additives, preservatives, artificial coloring, and added sugars that may exacerbate your symptoms. Moreover, you have the flexibility to choose fruits and vegetables that are gentle on digestion, helping to reduce uncomfortable symptoms like bloating and abdominal distension–two common and unpleasant issues associated with SIBO.

Another significant benefit of homemade juices is their ability to enhance your nutrient intake with ease. For individuals who have difficulty digesting solid foods, juices serve as excellent allies. They deliver concentrated amounts of vitamins, minerals, antioxidants, and other essential nutrients from fresh fruits and vegetables. Every glass becomes a powerhouse of nutrition that supports both overall health and your digestive system's functionality.

Hydration is another crucial aspect that homemade juices address. Staying properly hydrated is vital for mitigating SIBO symptoms, and juices made with water-rich fruits such as melon or pineapple offer a delicious way to achieve this. This approach delivers twofold benefits: keeping you well-hydrated while providing essential nutrients at the same time.

Furthermore, homemade juices have the unique advantage of removing insoluble fiber during the juicing process. For people with SIBO, insoluble fiber can be problematic, as it promotes fermentation and gas production within the gut, worsening symptoms. By offering nutrients without this type of fiber, juices provide a lighter, easier option to nourish your body without adding undue strain to your digestive system.

In summary, homemade juices are an effective and refreshing way to introduce essential nutrients into your diet, particularly if consuming solid foods is a challenge. For those with SIBO, carefully managing your diet can make a profound difference, and homemade juices are a versatile, health-enhancing tool that can support your digestive health while adding vibrant energy to your day.

Overall Health Benefits of Juices and Smoothies

Incorporating juices or smoothies into your diet can be an excellent choice for your health. Here are some of their most significant benefits:

‣ **Compliance with Recommended Fruit and Vegetable Intake**: Smoothies and shakes offer a practical and enjoyable way to meet the daily recommendation of five servings of fruits and vegetables. They provide a diverse range of essential nutrients that support optimal health and overall well-being.

‣ **Easy Assimilation and Digestion**: As liquid meals, smoothies and shakes are gentler on the digestive system and allow for quicker nutrient absorption. They are especially beneficial for individuals with digestive sensitivities or challenges.

‣ **Vitamin and Mineral Powerhouse**: Made from fresh fruits and vegetables, smoothies and shakes are rich sources of essential vitamins and minerals that promote the proper functioning of the body.

‣ **Detoxification and Cleansing**: Ingredients like leafy greens and natural antioxidants help flush out toxins, enhance cell health, and support effective internal cleansing.

‣ **Balancing Body pH**: By incorporating alkaline foods, smoothies and shakes play a key role in stabilizing the body's pH levels, aiding disease prevention and improving overall wellness.

‣ **Reduction of Inflammation**: Anti-inflammatory additions such as turmeric, ginger, and leafy greens can help minimize inflammation, fostering better health and increased comfort.

‣ **A Balanced Meal Replacement**: When combined with protein, healthy fats, and complex carbohydrates, smoothies become a nourishing and balanced meal replacement. They provide sustained energy and promote fullness throughout the day.

‣ **Supports Weight Management**: With their low-calorie yet nutrient-dense profiles, smoothies and shakes encourage healthy eating habits. They help manage appetite and support maintaining or achieving an ideal weight.

‣ **Enhances Skin Health**: Packed with skin-friendly vitamins like A and C from fresh ingredients, smoothies and shakes contribute to hydrated, radiant, and healthy skin.

‣ **Slows Cellular Aging**: The antioxidants in smoothie ingredients combat oxidative damage, protect cells, and help maintain a youthful appearance.

‣ **Boosts Energy and Vitality**: Smoothies made with superfoods provide a steady energy boost, helping you stay active, energized, and revitalized throughout the day.

In conclusion, smoothies and shakes are a nutritious, convenient, and versatile addition to your diet. Not only do they simplify the daily intake of fruits and vegetables, but they also provide a wide range of benefits for your overall health and well-being—all in a delicious and easy-to-enjoy form.

Homemade vs. Commercial Juices

Nowadays, identifying which foods truly benefit our health can be quite challenging. Supermarkets are overflowing with an extensive range of options, flaunting attractive packaging and clever designs that promise to be natural and healthy. While advertising and packaging often catch our attention, are we genuinely purchasing natural beverages made from fruits and vegetables? Do you know the key differences between homemade juices and industrial products? Are packaged products really as nutritious as they claim to be? Taking a few moments to carefully read ingredient labels and analyze their composition may uncover some surprising truths.

A few years ago, international regulations were established to define the standards that every fruit-based beverage must meet, specifying precise characteristics for each type of product. Below, we'll explore these distinctions and delve into the essential differences.

▸ Fruit Juice
Fruit juice is derived from fresh, chilled, or frozen fruits without undergoing any fermentation. It may contain separately extracted pulp and, in some cases, be blended with juice from various fruits. Labels are required to specify the composition in descending order, including the exact percentage of each fruit.

To prolong shelf life and eliminate the need for refrigeration, fruit juice is typically sterilized or pasteurized. Unfortunately, these processes result in significant nutrient loss, particularly impacting essential vitamins and enzymes. Moreover, the juice lacks the natural fiber found in whole fruits.

▸ Juice from Concentrates
Juice from concentrates is created by reconstituting dehydrated juice concentrates with water. Concentrates are produced by extracting natural juice through evaporation or other physical methods. During reconstitution, manufacturers may add aromas or pulp from similar fruits to partially restore flavor.

Though widely consumed, these juices suffer nutrient losses during production, including enzymes, vitamins, minerals, and the valuable fiber that characterizes natural fruit.

▸ Dehydrated or Powdered Fruit Juice
This product is manufactured by removing water from fruit to create a dry powder, which can later be rehydrated or sold in its dehydrated state. However, the dehydration process significantly diminishes its nutritional value, leading to the loss of enzymes, vitamins, minerals, and natural fiber.

▸ Fruit Nectar
Fruit nectar differs from pure juice as it is made using fruit concentrate, water, and added sugars or sweeteners. Its

nutritional value is considerably lower compared to natural fruit juices due to its inclusion of artificial additives to enhance flavor, color, or shelf life.

‣ Juice-Based Drinks

These beverages typically combine various fruits but contain minimal actual fruit juice. Often, they lack the essential nutrients derived from fruits, consisting largely of water, artificial aromas, colorings, and sweeteners.

‣ Milk-Infused Juice Drinks

Milk-infused juice drinks include fruit juice, often from concentrates, in very small proportions. They are mixed with milk, water, flavorings, and other ingredients. These beverages are not considered true juices, and any nutrients present are artificially added during manufacturing to compensate for losses incurred during processing.

‣ Vegetable and/or Greens Juice

Vegetable and greens juices are extracted from vegetables using specialized industrial methods, often with added pulp or pureed ingredients. They may also blend various vegetables to create balanced or palatable flavors.

To extend shelf life and eliminate refrigeration requirements, these juices undergo pasteurization or sterilization, which unfortunately reduces essential nutrients, including vitamins and phytonutrients. Additionally, they lack the natural fiber of whole vegetables and may include preservatives, salt, or flavor enhancers that compromise their nutritional profile.

‣ Commercial Smoothies

Commercial smoothies are typically prepared by blending fruits, vegetables, and greens—often using purees or concentrates—with water, milk, plant-based beverages, or similar liquids. Their thicker texture comes from a higher proportion of pulp or fiber-rich components.

To enhance taste, appearance, and shelf life, industrial smoothies usually contain added sugars, preservatives, colorings, and flavorings that alter their natural composition.

Moreover, they undergo pasteurization or thermal sterilization to allow room-temperature storage, further degrading their original nutrients and reducing their overall nutritional quality.

Advantages of Homemade Juices

After uncovering what commercial preparations truly contain, it becomes evident that making them at home offers numerous advantages. Here are the most significant ones:

‣ **Complete Control Over Ingredients**: Preparing your own juices allows you to ensure the quality of the ingredients you use. There are no unnecessary additives, no preservatives, and–most importantly–no unpleasant surprises.

‣ **Variety and Creativity**: You have the freedom to choose your favorite fruits and vegetables, experiment with unique combinations, or incorporate fresh, seasonal produce. This not only provides a burst of delicious flavors but also boosts your intake of essential nutrients.

‣ **Authentic Aroma and Flavor**: Homemade juices retain the genuine aroma and taste of fresh fruits and vegetables. There's truly nothing like enjoying a freshly made juice packed with natural freshness.

‣ **Maximum Nutrient Retention**: Vitamins, minerals, enzymes, antioxidants, and other nutrients remain intact when you prepare juices at home, significantly enhancing their health benefits.

‣ **Premium Quality Ingredients**: Choosing fresh, seasonal produce at its peak ripeness ensures optimal flavor and exceptional nutritional value.

‣ **Seasonal Food Benefits**: Consuming fruits and vegetables that are in season supports sustainability, is more cost-effective, and often results in better taste and nutritional quality.

‣ **Total Customization**: Whether using a juicer or blender, you can adjust the consistency of your juice to your liking–whether you prefer a light, clear juice or a thicker, fiber-rich option.

‣ **Kid-Friendly Option**: Homemade juices are an excellent way to incorporate fruits and vegetables into children's diets, especially for picky eaters. With creative flavors and fun presentations, you can make juices irresistible for kids.

In conclusion, smoothies and shakes are a nutritious, convenient, and versatile addition to your diet. Not only do they simplify the daily intake of fruits and vegetables, but they also provide a wide range of benefits for your overall health and well-being–all in a delicious and easy-to-enjoy form.

Possible Adverse Effects

If you suffer from **SIBO, gastritis, colitis, irritable bowel syndrome, or constipation**, it's essential to take certain precautions when preparing smoothies or juices. Following these recommendations will help you enjoy their benefits without worsening your symptoms:

‣ **Use a juicer instead of a blender**: For digestive health conditions, it's often better to use a juicer rather than a blender when making juices. Juicing removes most of the fiber from the ingredients, resulting in a smoother liquid that is gentler on your digestive system.

‣ **Moderate your fiber intake**: Although fiber is highly beneficial for overall health, excessive consumption can lead to gas, bloating, or constipation–especially for individuals with sensitive digestion. Be mindful of the fiber content in your smoothies by limiting ingredients like fruit pulp, seeds, and whole grains.

‣ **Introduce juices gradually**: If you're unsure how your body will react, start with small portions. This enables you to monitor their effects on your digestion and adjust the recipes to suit your specific needs.

▸ **Consume juices on an empty stomach**: Drinking juices on an empty stomach can maximize nutrient absorption and aid digestion. This approach minimizes the risk of digestive discomfort and helps you fully benefit from the juice's nutrients.

▸ **Tailor recipes to your personal needs**: Everyone's digestive system is unique, and responses to certain foods can vary greatly. Pay close attention to how your body reacts after consuming juices, and adapt ingredient combinations to best support your health and well-being.

When to Take Them

There are several effective ways to incorporate juices into your routine, depending on your goals and daily habits. Below are three recommended methods:

▸ **In the morning, on an empty stomach**: Begin your day with a carefully chosen juice recipe, consuming it before eating anything else. Drinking juice on an empty stomach enhances nutrient absorption and stimulates your digestive system, helping prepare it for the rest of the day.

▸ **On an empty stomach, before meals**: Enjoy a juice approximately 30 minutes before your main meals to maximize its benefits. This practice supports digestion and boosts nutrient absorption, promoting overall health and well-being.

▸ **Juice-based fasting**: Engage in a multi-day fast consisting exclusively of juices to achieve specific health objectives or to detoxify your body. Choose 2 to 3 recipes and consume them consistently throughout the day to stay nourished and energized.

Preparation Tips

Preparing fresh juices is an easy and nutritious way to make the most of the vitamins and minerals found in fruits and vegetables. To optimize the process and ensure safety, consider the following recommendations:

▸ **Choose organic ingredients**: Whenever possible, opt for organic fruits and vegetables. They provide cleaner, pesticide-free consumption and promote a healthier lifestyle.

▸ **Wash ingredients thoroughly**: Rinse all produce carefully to remove dirt, bacteria, and chemical residues. Trim any bruised, moldy, or damaged areas to prevent contamination.

▸ **Cut ingredients into smaller pieces**: Make blending easier by chopping fruits and vegetables into smaller, manageable chunks. This helps achieve a smoother texture and shortens preparation time.

▸ **Balance ingredients with low water content**: Fruits and vegetables with low water content, such as bananas and avocados, may require pre-mixing. Start with juicier ingredients to create a liquid base, then gradually add denser items for a cohesive blend.

▸ **Peel certain fruits appropriately**: Remove citrus rinds (like those from oranges and grapefruits), as their outer layers may contain toxins. However, keep the nutrient-rich white inner layer. Peel tropical fruits, such as papayas and kiwis, especially if they are grown in regions with less stringent chemical regulations.

▸ **Discard harmful seeds**: Remove seeds from apples, as they contain trace amounts of cyanide and are unsafe to consume. On the other hand, seeds from grapes, melons, lemons, and limes are safe and offer additional health benefits.

▸ **Incorporate stems and leaves mindfully**: Many stems and leaves are nutritious, but be cautious. Avoid toxic ones, such as carrot and rhubarb leaves, which can be harmful.

▸ **Drink your juice immediately**: Freshly prepared juice is best consumed right away to minimize nutrient loss and avoid oxidation. This ensures maximum freshness and health benefits.

▸ **Remove bitter celery leaves**: Bitter celery leaves can affect the flavor of your juice. Remove them before blending the stalks to create a more balanced and enjoyable taste.

Key Recommendations

Smoothies and shakes are an excellent, healthy alternative, but to get the most out of them, it's essential to keep certain aspects in mind. Below are some key recommendations:

▸ **Moderate fruit consumption**: Fruits are a fantastic source of nutrients but also contain fructose, a natural sugar that, when consumed excessively, can impact your health. Strive for balance by moderating your fruit intake throughout the day. Additionally, avoid eating fruits at night, as the body may metabolize them less efficiently during this time.

▸ **Choose seasonal fruits**: Seasonal fruits are often more nutrient-rich, flavorful, and cost-effective. By opting for fruits in season, you can enjoy their peak freshness and nutritional benefits while saving money.

▸ **Pick compatible combinations**: Not all fruits or ingredients blend well together. Research suitable pairings to create a smoothie or shake with balanced flavors and optimal nutritional value.

▸ **Use a moderate amount of ingredients**: The simplest smoothies are often the best. Avoid overloading them with excessive ingredients, which can lead to heavy textures or digestive discomfort. Stick to recommended recipes and be mindful of proportions.

▸ **Include leafy greens and vegetables**: Incorporate leafy greens, like spinach or kale, or vegetables, such as cucumber, to lower the glycemic index and boost your drink's nutrient profile. These additions make your smoothie both healthier and more satisfying.

▸ **Use natural sweeteners in moderation**: Enjoy the natural flavors of the ingredients, but if sweetening is necessary, choose options like raw honey or pure stevia. Use them sparingly to maintain a balanced nutritional profile.

▸ **Chew your drink**: Even liquid smoothies benefit from being "chewed." This simple habit stimulates the release of digestive enzymes, helping improve nutrient absorption and reducing discomfort like bloating or indigestion.

▸ **Store properly**: For the best results, consume smoothies or shakes fresh. If storing is needed, place them in a dark, airtight container in the refrigerator, or freeze individual portions for later use.

▸ **Make them fun and personalized**: Add an enjoyable twist by freezing smoothies in molds with fun shapes–an excellent way to turn a healthy drink into a delightful treat, especially for children.

These recommendations will help you make the most of your smoothies and shakes. While the recipes provided in this book are crafted to facilitate nutrient absorption, always remember that individual needs vary. Feel free to experiment with different combinations, tailor recipes to suit your tastes, and prioritize your health and well-being. Enjoy the journey to a healthier lifestyle!

Suggested Recipes

Here are several juice options carefully tailored for people managing SIBO:

▸ **Pineapple and ginger juice**
Ingredients: 1 cup fresh pineapple, 1 slice ginger, 1 cup water.
Preparation: Blend all ingredients in a blender until smooth. Drink immediately.

▸ **Spinach and strawberry smoothie**
Ingredients: 1 cup fresh spinach, 1 cup strawberries, 1 banana*, 1 cup coconut water.

Preparation: Blend all ingredients in a blender until smooth. Enjoy this refreshing smoothie.

Note*: Although green bananas tend to be better tolerated by some people with SIBO due to their lower fermentable sugar content, it is essential to remember that individual tolerance may vary. Some people may still experience bloating or abdominal discomfort due to the resistant fiber found in green bananas. It is always advisable to observe how your body reacts to the addition of green bananas and/or ripe bananas to recipes and adjust your intake accordingly.

‣ Carrot and beetroot juice
Ingredients: 2 carrots, 1 beetroot, 1 <u>green</u> apple*, 1/2 lemon (juice).
Preparation: Pass the carrots, beetroot, and apple through a juicer. Add the lemon juice and mix well. Drink immediately.

Note*: <u>Green</u> apples cause fewer adverse effects in people with SIBO than ripe apples. Green apples contain less fructose and fermentable carbohydrates, which may help reduce the likelihood of triggering unpleasant symptoms associated with SIBO.

‣ Cucumber and mint juice
Ingredients: 1 cucumber, a few leaves of fresh mint, 1 lemon (juice), 1 cup of water.
Preparation: Put the cucumber and mint leaves through a juice extractor. Add lemon juice and water. Mix well, then enjoy.

‣ Pineapple and coconut smoothie
Ingredients: 1 cup fresh pineapple, 1 cup coconut milk, 1 banana*, 1 tablespoon chia seeds.
Preparation: Blend all ingredients in a blender until smooth and creamy. Serve cold.

‣ Carrot, ginger, and turmeric juice
Ingredients: 2 carrots, 1 slice ginger, 1/2 teaspoon turmeric powder, 1/2 lemon (juice), 1 cup water.
Preparation: Pass the carrots and ginger through a juicer. Add

turmeric, lemon juice, and water. Mix well and drink.

‣ Apple and celery juice
Ingredients: 2 <u>green</u> apples*, 2 celery stalks, 1 small cucumber, 1/2 lemon (juice).

Preparation: Pass the green apples, celery, and cucumber through a juicer. Add the lemon juice and blend well. Enjoy this refreshing juice.

‣ Spinach and banana smoothie:
Ingredients: 2 cups fresh spinach, 1 ripe banana*, 1 tablespoon almond butter, 1 cup unsweetened almond milk.

Preparation: Blend all ingredients in a blender until smooth and creamy. Serve cold.

‣ Orange and carrot juice:
Ingredients: 3 oranges, 2 carrots, 1 small piece of ginger.

Preparation: Pass the oranges and carrots through a juicer. Add grated ginger and mix well. Drink immediately.

‣ Watermelon and mint juice:
Ingredients: 2 cups seedless watermelon, a few leaves of fresh mint, 1 lime (juice).

Preparation: Run the watermelon through a juice extractor. Add the finely chopped mint leaves and lime juice. Mix well, and enjoy this refreshing juice.

‣ Papaya and ginger smoothie:
Ingredients: 1 cup fresh papaya, 1 slice ginger, 1 cup unsweetened almond milk, 1 tablespoon flaxseed.

Preparation: Blend papaya, ginger, almond milk, and flax seeds until smooth. Serve and enjoy.

‣ Kale and cucumber green juice:
Ingredients: 2 cups kale, 1 cucumber, 1 <u>green</u> apple, 1/2 lemon (juice), 1 cup coconut water.

Preparation: Pass the kale, cucumber, and apple through a juicer. Add lemon juice and coconut water. Mix well and drink.

‣ Beetroot and carrot juice:
Ingredients: 1 beetroot, 2 carrots, 1 <u>green</u> apple, 1 small piece

of ginger.

Preparation: Pass the beetroot, carrots, and apple through a juicer. Add the grated ginger and mix well. Drink immediately.

▶ **Berry and almond smoothie:**

Ingredients: 1 cup mixed berries (strawberries, blueberries, raspberries), 1 banana*, 1 cup unsweetened almond milk, 1 tablespoon almond butter.

Preparation: Blend all ingredients in a blender until smooth and creamy. Serve and enjoy.

▶ **Pineapple, mint, and spinach juice:**

Ingredients: 1 cup fresh pineapple, a handful of fresh spinach, a few mint leaves, 1 lime (juice).

Preparation: Pass the pineapple, spinach, and mint through a juicer. Add the lime juice and mix well. Drink immediately.

Most people with SIBO generally tolerate the recommended juices well. However, since individual responses can vary, it's a good idea to monitor how you feel a few hours after consuming them. If you experience any discomfort, try introducing them gradually into your diet, ideally on an empty stomach.

Enjoy these tasty and nutritious options!

MEDICINAL PLANTS

"Nature is the wisest physician" (Hippocrates)

Since time immemorial, humanity has turned to the natural world for answers to its needs. Medicinal herbs, faithful companions on this journey, have generously shared their wisdom to ease ailments and enhance well-being. This ancient knowledge, carefully preserved through the ages, has found a renewed place in the modern world, offering a healthy and sustainable option to address today's challenges.

In a society increasingly conscious of the adverse effects of certain pharmaceutical treatments and the environmental toll of unsustainable practices, botanical remedies are experiencing a resurgence with renewed prominence. For those seeking a balanced, respectful lifestyle in harmony with the environment, these green treasures provide invaluable solutions. This revival not only reflects a growing interest in ecological approaches but also an evolution toward holistic care for both the body and the planet.

What makes these natural wonders truly extraordinary is the complexity of their compounds, capable of delivering antioxidant, anti-inflammatory, antibacterial, and antiviral properties, among others. Their potential ranges from alleviating everyday issues like sleeplessness or sluggish digestion to addressing conditions such as chronic stress or age-related ailments.

Beyond the ability to target specific concerns, these species serve as vital sources of micronutrients–vitamins, minerals, fiber, and antioxidants–that fortify the immune system and support long-term health. Incorporating them into dietary or self-care routines offers a simple, sustainable, and effective path toward illness prevention and enhanced overall wellness.

The botanical kingdom boasts remarkable diversity, featuring countless species uniquely suited to meet specific needs. Whether prepared as herbal teas, applied as balms or tinctures, or utilized in the form of essential oils, their applications are as versatile as they are effective, seamlessly fitting into various lifestyles.

More than mere remedies, these natural allies inspire us to reconnect with the world around us. Harnessing their benefits requires respect for environmental rhythms and a deeper appreciation for our planet's ecosystems. Each herb or extract serves as a tangible reminder of our connection to the living world, fostering a sense of harmony that transcends the physical and nurtures the spiritual.

In addition to their myriad health benefits, plant-based solutions stand out for their accessibility and practical versatility. Many species grow abundantly in wild habitats or can be easily cultivated in home gardens, offering an affordable, sustainable alternative. In a global context marked by economic inequalities, these wellness allies provide inclusive options to complement–or even replace–costly interventions.

Over the centuries, knowledge of these natural solutions has been carefully preserved through oral traditions and written records. This heritage, rooted in deep respect for biodiversity, has been bolstered by modern science, validating the effects of their active compounds and shedding light on their mechanisms of action. It represents a powerful synergy between tradition and innovation, broadening the therapeutic applications of these botanical marvels.

However, unlocking their full potential requires responsible use. Every human body is unique, and while these species possess well-documented therapeutic properties, they are not without risks. Misuse or interactions with conventional medications can lead to adverse effects. Therefore, obtaining accurate and reliable information is essential to ensure safe and effective usage.

One particularly fascinating aspect is how the components within a plant work in unison. Whole extracts, resulting from this intricate interaction, often produce more balanced and holistic effects compared to isolated compounds. Molecules interact in complementary ways, maximizing benefits while reducing potential side effects. Conversely, isolated active principles can provide concentrated solutions but may carry an increased risk of adverse effects on the body.

The innate harmony of these botanical wonders highlights one of biodiversity's greatest gifts–balance. Whole extracts are celebrated for their gentleness and ability to integrate seamlessly with the body's natural processes. On the other hand, synthesized compounds strive for potency, often at the expense of stability. The synergistic interaction between molecular components amplifies therapeutic benefits while limiting potential downsides, making them a choice deeply aligned with human needs.

Ultimately, medicinal plants transcend their role as therapeutic tools–they bridge ancestral wisdom and scientific innovation. They remind us that the health of our bodies and the well-being of our planet are profoundly interconnected. By safeguarding this invaluable legacy, we nurture not only our own health but also that of future generations, renewing the delicate balance between humanity and nature.

Essential Information

Although plants are natural in origin, they should not be considered entirely harmless. Their active compounds may cause adverse effects or trigger allergies in certain individuals.

Occasional consumption of an infusion is unlikely to cause harm. However, excessive, prolonged, or frequent use may result in discomfort, allergic reactions, or even toxicity.

Tolerance to natural remedies varies greatly among individuals. If you are pregnant, breastfeeding, or managing conditions such as chronic illnesses, allergies, kidney or liver insufficiency, cancer, or undergoing medical treatment, it is crucial to refer to the section titled "**Side Effects, Contraindications, and Interactions**" before using them. This section provides essential information on potential risks, enabling you to make informed and responsible decisions.

Guidelines for Care with Herbal Remedies

For best results, continue using the remedies until your symptoms have completely disappeared. The treatment duration will vary depending on factors like the severity of your condition, how it progresses, your personal commitment, and other important influences.

Keep in mind that some plants or herbal remedies are not suited for continuous or long-term use. In such cases, you will always find specific instructions that address this.

While following the guidelines for the remedies, it is just as important to focus on the underlying causes of your symptoms. To better understand the root of your health concerns, I recommend referring to the first chapter of this book, specifically the section titled "Causes," where you'll discover essential insights into tackling the problem at its source.

Finally, remember that patience is vital. A condition that has lingered for months or years cannot be resolved in just a few days. Stay committed, persevere, and always prioritize your health and well-being.

Medicinal Plants and SIBO

In the sequential treatment outlined in "Supplements for SIBO: A 9-Step Plan", the incorporation of medicinal plants becomes a key focus starting from Step 5. Ideally, the process begins with addressing bacterial overgrowth using the nutritional supplements recommended in the earlier stages. Once Step 4 is completed, the medicinal plants discussed below can be introduced.

These plants provide a holistic approach to managing this condition. Each one contains phytochemicals–natural compounds with therapeutic properties that can effectively relieve symptoms. Let's explore their benefits:

‣ **Carminative properties**: Plants with these properties help alleviate bloating and discomfort caused by intestinal gas accumulation.

Peppermint, ginger, and fennel seeds are the three highly recommended plants with this attribute.

‣ **Anti-inflammatory properties**: Intestinal inflammation plays a significant role in SIBO. These plants' capacity to diminish inflammation helps mitigate symptoms and support gut healing.

The three highly recommended plants are turmeric, ginger, and chamomile.

‣ **Antispasmodic properties**: These properties aid in calming intestinal spasms and alleviating associated discomfort.

The three most recommended plants are peppermint, lavender, and chamomile.

‣ **Immunomodulatory properties**: Certain medicinal plants are recognized for their capacity to modulate the immune response, which is pertinent as immune dysfunction is implicated in SIBO development. These plants contain bioactive compounds that impact immune function, either by bolstering the immune system or by assisting in regulating overactive immune responses commonly observed in the context of SIBO.

The three recommended plants are licorice, turmeric, and ginger

‣ **Peristaltic properties**: Research has also explored the impact of medicinal plants on intestinal motility. Intestinal motility refers to the movement of gastrointestinal tract muscles that facilitate food passage through the digestive system. Proper intestinal peristalsis prevents bacterial overgrowth in the small intestine, which is beneficial in SIBO.

The three recommended plants are turmeric, peppermint, and aloe vera.

‣ **Prebiotic properties**: The potential of specific medicinal plants to enhance gut microbiota health and balance is an area of growing research interest. Utilizing these plants can address gut dysbiosis, an imbalance in microbiota composition. Some plants contain prebiotic compounds that foster the growth of beneficial bacteria in the gut, which is crucial for counteracting the proliferation of pathogenic bacteria associated with SIBO.

The three recommended plants are chicory root, burdock root, and dandelion.

‣ **Astringent properties**: Certain plants possess properties that aid in restoring the integrity of the intestinal barrier and reducing intestinal permeability. This is crucial in SIBO, where the intestinal lining may be compromised. A leaky gut is a prevalent issue in this condition and requires attention.

Recommended plants include barberry and black raspberry.

‣ **Analgesic properties**: Compounds in select plants help alleviate the sensation of abdominal pain and discomfort, common symptoms in individuals with SIBO.

The three recommended plants are chamomile, peppermint, and valerian.

‣ **Hepatic properties**: Certain plants exhibit beneficial effects on liver function, facilitating detoxification and proper nutrient metabolism, which is vital in the comprehensive management of SIBO.

The three recommended plants are milk thistle, dandelion,

and turmeric.

▸ **Restorative properties**: Specific medicinal plants can address nutritional imbalances and malabsorption linked to SIBO. These plants contain nutrients and compounds that enhance digestion and nutrient absorption, benefiting people with SIBO who have nutritional deficiencies.

The three recommended plants are echinacea, Siberian ginseng, and ashwagandha.

▸ **Antioxidant properties**: Certain medicinal plants contain compounds with antioxidant properties, which are beneficial for managing SIBO. Oxidative stress contributes to inflammation and tissue damage, and the antioxidants in these plants help neutralize free radicals and safeguard cells in the small intestine from harm.

The three recommended plants are rosemary, turmeric, and green tea.

▸ **Neuroprotective properties**: Certain medicinal plants encompass compounds with neuroprotective properties that positively impact communication between the brain and the gut. This is pertinent as SIBO has frequently been observed to affect the functionality of the enteric nervous system or "second brain."

The enteric nervous system comprises an intricate network of millions of neurons located in the gastrointestinal tract. These neurons govern various digestive functions, including intestinal motility, enzyme secretion, and gut permeability. Additionally, this 'second brain' plays a pivotal role in communicating with the central nervous system and regulating local immune responses in the gut.

The recommended plants are bacopa and ashwagandha.

▸ **Relaxing properties**: Some plants contain compounds with relaxing properties that help reduce stress and anxiety, which can impact the symptomatology of SIBO.

The three recommended plants are chamomile, lavender, and valerian.

‣ **Hormone-regulating properties**: Hormonal imbalances often present in individuals with SIBO can also be addressed. Certain medicinal plants contain phytohormones and compounds that aid in regulating hormonal balance in the body.

The three recommended plants are licorice, nettle, and dong quai (Angelica sinensis).

‣ **Detoxifying or depurative properties**: Specific medicinal plants promote body detoxification, aiding in the elimination of toxins and unwanted compounds that may accumulate due to SIBO and bowel dysfunction.

The three recommended plants are turmeric, milk thistle, and dandelion root.

‣ **Nutritional properties**: Moreover, medicinal plants serve as a natural source of nutrients, including vitamins, minerals, antioxidants, and phytonutrients. These prove beneficial for individuals with SIBO who experience nutritional deficiencies due to malabsorption and gut microbiota imbalances.

The three recommended plants are ginger, chamomile, and mint

‣ **Adaptogenic properties**: Certain medicinal plants contain compounds with adaptogenic properties. These properties assist the body in adapting to and recovering from stress, which is advantageous for individuals with SIBO who face physiological and emotional stress as part of their condition.

The three recommended plants are ashwagandha, rhodiola, and Siberian ginseng.

It is critical to emphasize that the use of medicinal plants does not replace conventional medical treatments prescribed by your specialist. However, they can effectively complement these treatments, providing additional support for comprehensive health care.

In the context of SIBO, medicinal plants can address several key aspects. Their benefits include relieving gastrointestinal symptoms and abdominal discomfort, improving the health and permeability of the intestinal lining, supporting liver function, optimizing digestion and nutrient absorption, and restoring balance to the intestinal microbiota. Additionally, they promote hormonal regulation, aid in the body's detoxification processes, modulate the immune response, and contribute to stress adaptation and emotional well-being. Furthermore, they help prevent complications, offering an integrative approach to the complementary treatment of SIBO.

In the following section, titled "Effective Plants for Managing SIBO," we will explore various plant-based options and their potential benefits.

Effective Plants for Managing SIBO

Presented below is a selection of plants renowned for their effectiveness in managing symptoms associated with this intestinal disorder. The information provided includes their properties, methods of preparation–such as infusions–other possible uses, and recommended dosages. Their scientific names are included in parentheses to ensure accurate identification, particularly as some plants may have different common names depending on the region or country.

It is essential to remember that each individual is unique and may experience this condition differently. Therefore, you should select the plants that best address your specific symptoms and the imbalances you wish to correct.

Aloe vera (Aloe barbadensis)

▸ **Benefits**

Aloe vera benefits bacterial overgrowth in the small intestine due to its antimicrobial, anti-inflammatory, and healing properties. It promotes intestinal health and balances the microbiota, thereby aiding in the reduction of unwanted bacterial growth in the small intestine.

▸ **Plant preparation and dosage**
The gel extracted directly from the plant's leaves can be used to prepare aloe vera. Mix one teaspoon of aloe gel in a glass of water and consume it before meals. While dosages may vary, it is generally recommended to commence with a small amount to assess tolerance and increase gradually if necessary.

▸ **Aloe Vera capsules or tablets and dosage**
Aloe vera is also available in capsule or tablet form. The recommended dosage is 100-300 mg daily, divided into 2 or 3 doses.

Ashwagandha (Withania somnifera)

▸ **Benefits**
Ashwagandha is an adaptogenic herb that can help with SIBO. Some potential advantages include its ability to reduce inflammation, balance the gut microbiota, and strengthen the immune system, ultimately enhancing overall gastrointestinal health.

▸ **Infusion preparation and dosage**
The dried and ground roots of the plant can be utilized to prepare an Ashwagandha infusion. Add a teaspoon of the root to a cup of hot water, steep for a few minutes, strain, and then consume. Aim to drink 1-2 cups per day, preferably with food.

▸ **Ashwagandha capsules or tablets and dosage**
Ashwagandha is also available in capsule or tablet form, containing extract from the plant's root. The suggested dose is 200-500 mg, twice daily. It is advisable to take it with food to enhance absorption and minimize any potential gastric irritation.

Bacopa (Bacopa monnieri)

▸ **Benefits**
Bacopa monnieri is an herbaceous plant with potential properties for enhancing gut health. Some reported benefits

include its ability to reduce inflammation, promote a balanced gut microbiota, and strengthen the immune system, all of which are advantageous for addressing bacterial overgrowth in the small intestine.

▸ Infusion preparation and dosage

The dried and crushed leaves of the Bacopa plant can be used to prepare an infusion. Add a teaspoon of leaves to a cup of hot water, steep for a few minutes, strain, and then consume. Take 1-2 times daily, preferably with food to aid absorption.

▸ Capsules or tablets and dosage

Bacopa is also available in capsule or tablet form, containing plant extract. The recommended dose is approximately 200-500 mg, divided into two doses. It is recommended to take it with food to enhance absorption and reduce the risk of stomach upset.

Barberry (Berberis vulgaris)

▸ Benefits

Barberry benefits individuals with SIBO due to its natural anti-microbial properties, which help regulate bacterial overgrowth in the area and support a healthy balance in gut flora.

▸ Infusion preparation and dosage

The dried and chopped bark of the barberry plant can be utilized to prepare a barberry infusion. Add a teaspoon of bark to a cup of hot water, steep for a few minutes, strain, and then consume. Aim to drink 2-3 cups daily, preferably before meals, to aid digestion.

▸ Barberry capsules or tablets and dosage

Barberry is also available in capsule or tablet form. Take one or two capsules containing 300-900 mg twice daily before meals for optimal results.

Burdock (Arctium lappa)

> **Benefits**

Burdock root is renowned for its medicinal properties and offers benefits for SIBO. Some advantages include its ability to promote gastrointestinal health, reduce inflammation, and serve as a prebiotic to foster a healthy balance in the gut microbiota.

> **Infusion preparation and dosage**

The dried and chopped root of the burdock plant can be utilized to prepare a burdock root infusion. To prepare it, add a teaspoon of the root to a cup of hot water, steep for a few minutes, strain, and then consume. Aim to drink one or two cups a day, preferably before meals.

> **Burdock root capsules or tablets and dosage**

Burdock root extract is also available in capsule or tablet form. The recommended dose is 400 to 1,800 mg per day, divided into two doses. It is advisable to take it before meals for enhanced efficacy in treating SIBO.

Chamomile (Matricaria chamomilla)

> **Benefits**

It is renowned for its soothing and anti-inflammatory properties, which provide gastrointestinal health benefits. It helps alleviate inflammation in the gastrointestinal tract, reduces stomach upset, improves digestion, and promotes a healthy balance in the gut microbiota. These effects benefit bacterial overgrowth in the small intestine by creating a more favorable intestinal environment.

> **Infusion preparation and dosage**

Dried chamomile flowers can be used to prepare chamomile tea. Add a teaspoon of flowers to a cup of hot water, allow it to steep for a few minutes, strain, and then drink. Aim to drink 2-3 cups daily, preferably after meals, to aid digestion.

> **Chamomile capsules or tablets and dosage**

Depending on the specific product's concentration, the recommended dose is 400 to 1,500 mg per day, divided into two or three doses after meals.

Chicory (Cichorium intybus)

‣ Benefits

Chicory's inulin content is advantageous for individuals with SIBO. Inulin is a prebiotic fiber that fosters the growth of beneficial bacteria in the gut, balancing the gut microbiota and enhancing digestion.

‣ Infusion preparation and dosage

The roasted and ground root of the chicory plant can be used to prepare a chicory infusion. To prepare it, add a teaspoon of chicory root to a cup of hot water, steep for a few minutes, strain, and then consume. Aim to drink 2-3 cups daily, preferably before meals, to assist digestion.

‣ Capsules or tablets and dosage

Chicory is also available in capsule or tablet form. The dosage for SIBO may vary, but it is generally advised to take one or two capsules containing 300 to 1,000 mg two or three times a day. It is recommended that the capsules be ingested before meals to prepare the digestive system.

Dandelion (Taraxacum officinale)

‣ Benefits

Dandelion is a plant traditionally used for its medicinal properties, including benefits for gut health. It can be a natural prebiotic, promote digestion, reduce inflammation, and support liver health. Thus, it positively influences the balance of the gut microbiota and addresses bacterial overgrowth in the small intestine.

‣ Infusion preparation and dosage

The plant's dried leaves can be used to prepare a dandelion infusion. Add a teaspoon of dandelion leaves to a cup of hot water, steep for a few minutes, strain, and then drink. Consume 2 cups a day, preferably after meals.

‣ Dandelion capsules or tablets and dosage

Dandelion is available in capsule or tablet form, containing plant extract. The recommended dose typically ranges from 400 to 1,900 mg per day, divided into two or three doses. It is advisable to take it with food to improve absorption and minimize any stomach upset.

Echinacea (Echinacea purpurea)

▶ **Benefits**

Echinacea is a plant recognized for its immunomodulatory and anti-inflammatory properties. It boosts the immune system, reduces inflammation, and supports overall gastro-intestinal health. These effects particularly benefit SIBO, balancing the gut microbiota and enhancing the body's natural defenses.

▶ **Infusion preparation and dosage**

The roots or aerial parts of the plant can be used to prepare an echinacea infusion. Add a teaspoon of echinacea to a cup of hot water, steep for a few minutes, strain, and then drink. It is recommended to consume one or two cups a day, preferably after meals.

▶ **Echinacea capsules or tablets and dosage**

Echinacea is also available in capsule or tablet form, containing plant extract. The suggested dose ranges from 200-1,100 mg daily, divided into 2 or 3 doses. It is advisable to take it with food to improve absorption and reduce the likelihood of stomach upset.

Dong quai (Angelica sinensis)

▶ **Benefits**

Dong Quai is an herb used in traditional Chinese medicine with beneficial gastrointestinal health properties. It helps reduce inflammation, improve digestion, and balance the intestinal microbiota, which is helpful for bacterial overgrowth in the small intestine.

▶ **Infusion preparation and dosage**

The plant's dried roots can be used to prepare an infusion of Dong Quai. Add a teaspoon of Dong Quai root to a cup of hot water and let it steep for a few minutes before straining and drinking. Take one or two cups a day, preferably before meals.

> ‣ **Dong Quai capsules or tablets and dosage**

Dong Quai is also available in capsule or tablet form. It contains an extract from the plant's root. Taking 400 to 1,900 mg per day is recommended, divided into two doses. It is advisable to take it with food to improve absorption and minimize stomach upset.

Fennel (Foeniculum vulgare)

> ‣ **Benefits**

Fennel seeds are renowned for their carminative and digestive properties. They help relieve bloating, enhance digestion, and reduce inflammation in the gastrointestinal tract. These effects particularly benefit bacterial overgrowth in the small intestine, fostering a more balanced and healthy intestinal environment.

> ‣ **Infusion preparation and dosage**

To prepare a fennel seed infusion, steep one teaspoon of fennel seeds in a cup of hot water for a few minutes before straining and drinking. Consuming fennel seed infusion after meals can help alleviate digestive symptoms. Aim to drink one to two cups daily, before or after meals.

Fennel seed capsules or tablets and dosage

Fennel seeds are also available in capsule or tablet form, containing seed extract. The recommended daily dose is typically 400-500 mg, divided into two or three doses. The seeds can be taken before or after meals.

Ginger (Zingiber officinale)

> ‣ **Benefits**

Ginger is renowned for its anti-inflammatory and digestive properties. It reduces inflammation in the gastrointestinal tract, alleviates stomach upset, improves digestion, and promotes a healthy balance in the gut microbiota. These effects are advantageous for SIBO by cultivating a more favorable gut environment and assisting in the digestive process.

> ‣ **Infusion preparation and dosage**

To prepare a ginger infusion, add a slice of fresh ginger to a cup of hot water, steep for a few minutes, and then drink. Aim to consume 2 or 3 cups daily, before or after meals.

▸ **Ginger capsules or tablets and dosage**
Ginger root extract is also available in capsule or tablet form. The recommended dose is 500 to 2,500 mg per day, divided into two or three doses. Depending on individual tolerance, it can be taken before or after meals.

Green tea (Camellia sinensis)

▸ **Benefits**
Green tea is known for its antioxidant and anti-inflammatory properties, as well as its overall health benefits. It has beneficial effects on gastrointestinal health by promoting healthy gut microbiota, reducing inflammation in the digestive tract, and improving digestion. These effects benefit SIBO by balancing the gut microbiota and promoting a healthy gut environment.

▸ **Infusion preparation and dosage**
To make a green tea infusion, boil water and pour it over the green tea leaves in a cup. Steep for 2 to 3 minutes, strain the leaves, and enjoy your brew. Consume 2 cups daily, in the morning and lunchtime between meals, to avoid interference with iron absorption or other nutrients.

▸ **Capsules or tablets and dosage**
The usual daily dose is 150 to 400 mg of green tea extract. It can be taken once or twice a day, before or after meals.

Note: Green tea contains caffeine, so it is recommended that you limit your consumption if you are sensitive to caffeine or have a caffeine-related issue.

Lavender (Lavandula angustifolia)

▸ **Benefits**
Lavender is renowned for its relaxing and calming properties, but also offers gastrointestinal health benefits. It reduces inflammation in the gastrointestinal tract, alleviates stomach upset, and promotes overall digestive health. These

effects can potentially benefit SIBO by fostering a more balanced gut environment.

‣ **Infusion preparation and dosage**
Dried lavender flowers can be used to prepare a lavender infusion. To prepare it, add a teaspoon of lavender flowers to a cup of hot water, allow it to steep for a few minutes, strain, and then drink. Consume one or two cups a day, preferably after meals.

‣ **Lavender capsules or tablets and dosage**
The typical daily dose is 50-140 mg, divided into two doses. It can be taken before or after meals, depending on individual tolerance and preference.

Licorice (Glycyrrhiza glabra)

‣ **Benefits**
Licorice is a plant with anti-inflammatory and antioxidant properties traditionally used for medicinal purposes. It offers gastrointestinal health benefits by helping to reduce inflammation in the digestive tract, promoting healthy intestinal mucosa, and balancing the intestinal microbiota.

‣ **Infusion preparation and dosage**
Boil water and pour over 1-2 teaspoons of dried licorice root. Let it steep for 5 to 10 minutes, strain, and drink 1-3 times a day, preferably before meals, to help stimulate digestion and soothe the gastrointestinal system.

‣ **Capsules or tablets and dosage**
Licorice capsules, tinctures, or extracts can also be taken if preferred. In capsule or tablet form, the typical daily dose can range from 100 mg to 500 mg, divided into one or two doses. It can be taken before or after meals, following specific product instructions.

Milk thistle (Silybum marianum)

‣ **Benefits**
Milk thistle, also known as silymarin, is a plant with hepatoprotective and antioxidant properties that benefit

intestinal health. It helps protect the liver and positively impacts gastrointestinal health by reducing the body's toxic burden.

▸ **Infusion preparation and dosage**
The crushed seeds of the plant can be used to prepare a milk thistle infusion. Add a teaspoon of milk thistle seeds to a cup of hot water, steep for a few minutes, strain, and then consume. Drink one cup one to two times a day before meals.

▸ **Milk thistle capsules or tablets and dosage**
Milk thistle is also available in capsule or tablet form, containing an extract from the plant's seeds. Taking 140-700 mg daily is recommended, divided into two doses. It is advisable to take it before meals for improved absorption and effectiveness in treating SIBO.

Nettle (Urtica dioica)

▸ **Benefits**
Nettle is a plant known for its anti-inflammatory and antioxidant properties. It helps reduce inflammation in the gastrointestinal tract, promotes healthy intestinal mucosa, and balances the intestinal microbiota.

▸ **Infusion preparation and dosage**
To prepare a nettle infusion, add a teaspoon of dried nettle leaves to a cup of hot water, allow it to steep for a few minutes, strain, and then drink. Drinking it two or three times a day, preferably before meals, is advisable to help stimulate digestion.

▸ **Capsules or tablets and dosage**
The recommended dose is 500 to 1,000 mg, divided into 1 or 2 doses. It can be taken before or after meals.

Peppermint (Mentha)

▸ **Benefits**
Peppermint is renowned for its digestive and cooling properties, aiding in relieving stomach upset, reducing inflammation in the gastrointestinal tract, improving digestion, and

promoting a more balanced gut environment. These effects are beneficial for SIBO by supporting overall digestive health and gut microbiota.

‣ Infusion preparation and dosage
Mint tea can be prepared using fresh or dried mint leaves. To prepare it, add a teaspoon of mint leaves to a cup of hot water, allow it to steep for a few minutes, strain, and then drink. Aim to consume two cups a day, either before or after meals.

‣ Peppermint capsules or tablets and dosage
The suggested dose is 150-300 mg per day in one or two doses. It can be taken before or after meals, depending on preference and tolerance.

Rhodiola (Rhodiola rosea)

‣ Benefits
Rhodiola is a plant with adaptogenic and anti-inflammatory properties that benefit gastrointestinal health. Rhodiola helps reduce inflammation, balance gut microbiota, and promote digestive health.

‣ Infusion preparation and dosage
To prepare a Rhodiola infusion, boil water. Place one teaspoon of Rhodiola root or dried herb in a cup, pour in the hot water, and let the infusion steep for about 10-15 minutes to release the active compounds into the water. Strain the infusion. The suggested daily intake is one to two times before meals, preferably in the morning and midday.

‣ Capsules or tablets and dosage
Rhodiola can be taken as capsules, liquid extracts, or tinctures. The dose in capsule or tablet form ranges from 100 to 500 mg daily, taken in one or two doses, preferably in the morning and midday before meals.

Rosemary (Rosmarinus officinalis)

‣ Benefits
Rosemary is an aromatic herb with antioxidant and anti-inflammatory properties that have beneficial effects on overall

gastrointestinal health. It reduces inflammation, promotes intestinal mucosal health, and balances the gut microbiota. These effects are helpful for bacterial overgrowth by promoting a more balanced gut environment.

> ▸ **Infusion preparation and dosage**

Boil water, place 1 teaspoon of dried rosemary in a cup, pour hot water over the rosemary, cover, steep for 5-10 minutes, strain, and drink 1-2 times daily. It can be taken before or after meals to help stimulate digestion and relieve stomach upset.

> ▸ **Capsules or tablets and dosage**

Rosemary can be taken as an infusion, tincture, or capsule. The dose in capsule or tablet form ranges from 400 mg to 900 mg a day, taken in one or two doses before or after meals.

Siberian ginseng (Eleutherococcus senticosus)

> ▸ **Benefits**

Siberian ginseng, also known as Eleutherococcus, is an adaptogenic herb with advantageous properties for gastrointestinal health. It can help reduce inflammation, strengthen the immune system, and promote a healthy balance in the gut microbiota, which is beneficial for SIBO.

> ▸ **Infusion preparation and dosage**

The plant's dried roots can be used to prepare a Siberian ginseng infusion. Add a teaspoon of the root to a cup of hot water, steep for a few minutes, strain, and then drink. To aid digestion, consume 1-2 cups daily, preferably before meals.

> ▸ **Siberian ginseng capsules or tablets and dosage**

Siberian ginseng is also available in capsule or tablet form, containing plant extract. It is recommended to take 200-1,100 mg per day, divided into two or three doses. It is preferable to take it before meals to maximize its benefits for digestion and the gastrointestinal system.

Turmeric (Curcuma longa)

> ▸ **Benefits**

Turmeric is a spice with anti-inflammatory and antioxidant properties. It benefits gut health by reducing inflammation, balancing the gut microbiota, and promoting overall digestive health.

▸ Infusion preparation and dosage

Either freshly grated root or turmeric powder can be used to prepare a turmeric infusion. To prepare it, add a teaspoon of turmeric powder to a cup of hot water, allow it to steep for a few minutes, and then drink. Consume a cup 1-2 times daily, preferably after meals, to aid digestion and reduce inflammation.

▸ Turmeric capsules or tablets and dosage

Turmeric is commonly consumed in capsule or tablet form. A typical daily dose ranges from 400 to 1,900 mg, divided into two or three doses. It is advisable to take it with food to enhance absorption and minimize potential stomach upset.

Valerian (Valeriana officinalis)

▸ Benefits

Valerian is a plant known for its sedative and calming properties. Its relaxing effects indirectly benefit gastrointestinal health by reducing stress and anxiety, as these emotions often negatively impact digestive function and the balance of gut microbiota.

▸ Infusion preparation and dosage

To prepare a valerian infusion, add one teaspoon of valerian root to a cup of hot water, let it steep for a few minutes, strain, and then drink. It is recommended to take it once or twice a day, preferably in the afternoon and/or evening before bed, as it can cause drowsiness.

▸ Capsules or tablets and dosage

The typical daily dose ranges from 200 mg to 500 mg. It can be divided into one or two doses, the last taken before bedtime or after meals.

Herbal Remedy Recipes

While the plants listed above are effective on their own, their properties can be significantly amplified when combined properly. Here are some especially effective combinations:

▸ **Phytotherapy Recipe No. 1**: *Digestive infusion*
- 1 teaspoon of ginger root
- 1 teaspoon of mint leaves
- 1 teaspoon of fennel seeds

Preparation: Mix the herbs in a cup of hot water. Steep for 5-10 minutes, strain, and drink before or after meals to aid digestion.

▸ **Phytotherapy Recipe No. 2**: *Anti-inflammatory Infusion*
- 1 teaspoon of turmeric powder
- 1 teaspoon of ginger root
- 1 teaspoon of mint leaves

Preparation: Mix the herbs in a cup of hot water. Steep for 5-10 minutes, strain, and drink to help reduce inflammation and promote digestive health.

▸ **Phytotherapy Recipe No. 3**: *Liver Tonic*
- 1 teaspoon of turmeric powder
- 1 teaspoon of milk thistle
- 1 teaspoon of licorice powder

Preparation: Mix the herbs in a cup of hot water. Steep for 5-10 minutes, strain, and drink as a liver tonic once daily to support liver function.

▸ **Phytotherapy Recipe No. 4**: *Soothing Infusion*
- 1 teaspoon of chamomile
- 1 teaspoon of licorice root
- 1 teaspoon of nettle leaves

Preparation: Mix the herbs in a cup of hot water. Steep for 5-10 minutes, strain, and drink before bedtime to help calm the digestive system and promote relaxation.

▸ **Phytotherapy Recipe No. 5**: *Digestive Infusion*
- 1 teaspoon of coriander seeds
- 1 teaspoon of mint leaves
- 1 teaspoon of licorice root

Preparation: Mix the herbs in a cup of hot water. Steep for 5-10 minutes, strain, and drink after meals to promote digestion and relieve stomach upset.

▸ **Phytotherapy Recipe No. 6**: *Anti-inflammatory Infusion*
- 1 teaspoon of turmeric powder
- 1 teaspoon of nettle leaves
- 1 teaspoon of ginger root

Preparation: Mix the herbs in a cup of hot water. Steep for 5-10 minutes, strain, and drink throughout the day to help reduce inflammation and support digestive health.

▸ **Phytotherapy Recipe No. 7**: *Liver and Digestive Tonic*
- 1 teaspoon of dandelion
- 1 teaspoon of artichoke leaves
- 1 teaspoon of ginger root

Preparation: Mix the herbs in a cup of hot water. Steep for 5-10 minutes, strain, and drink before meals to aid digestion and support liver function.

▸ **Phytotherapy Recipe No. 8**: *Soothing Infusion for the Digestive System*
- 1 teaspoon of licorice root
- 1 teaspoon of mint leaves
- 1 teaspoon of ginger root

Preparation: Mix the herbs in a cup of hot water. Steep for 5-10 minutes, strain, and drink to help soothe the digestive system and relieve stomach upset.

▸ **Phytotherapy Recipe No. 9**: Balancing Infusion
- 1 teaspoon of chamomile
- 1 teaspoon of milk thistle
- 1 teaspoon of licorice root

Preparation: Mix the herbs in a cup of hot water. Steep for 5-10 minutes, strain, and drink throughout the day to help balance digestive function and support liver health.

Before trying any of these recipes, it is essential to carefully review the potential side effects, contraindications, and interactions with medications, all of which are thoroughly detailed in the final section of this chapter. Be sure to remove or replace any plant that may not be appropriate for your specific situation.

Side Effects, Contraindications, and Interactions

In this section, the recommended medicinal plants are organized alphabetically for easy reference and accessibility. Before using any of them, it is crucial to thoroughly review the detailed information provided. This becomes even more important if you have a medical condition, a specific health issue, or are undergoing treatment, as there may be potential incompatibilities or side effects when combined with certain medications or health circumstances.

Making informed decisions is essential to minimizing unnecessary risks. Always keep in mind that your safety and well-being should remain the top priority when it comes to managing your health.

Aloe vera (Aloe barbadensis)

‣ **Side effects**: It may cause gastrointestinal irritation, such as diarrhea and cramps. Some individuals may also experience skin allergies, like redness or itching. In high doses, aloe vera can act as a laxative, leading to electrolyte imbalances.

‣ **Contraindications**: Aloe vera may stimulate uterine contractions during pregnancy. It should also be avoided by individuals with kidney, heart, or gastrointestinal conditions and those with known allergies.

‣ **Interactions**: Aloe vera may interact with diuretics and diabetes medications, potentially intensifying their effects. It may also interact with drugs that impact the heart, such as digoxin.

Ashwagandha (Withania somnifera)

‣ **Side effects**: Ashwagandha is generally well tolerated; however, in high doses, it may cause stomach upset and diarrhea in some individuals.

‣ **Contraindications**: Ashwagandha may further reduce blood pressure, so caution should be exercised in individuals with low blood pressure. It is also advisable to avoid its use during pregnancy and lactation.

‣ **Interactions**: Ashwagandha may interact with medications that affect blood pressure, diabetes, and the immune system. If you are taking any medications, it is crucial to consult a doctor or pharmacist before using them.

Bacopa (Bacopa monnieri)

‣ **Side effects**: It is generally safe, but in some instances, it may cause stomach upset, nausea, diarrhea, fatigue, or dry mouth.

‣ **Contraindications**: Caution should be exercised in people with heart problems, stomach ulcers, thyroid disorders, or in pregnant or breastfeeding women.

‣ **Interactions**: It may interact with thyroid medications, sedatives, antidepressants, and blood pressure medications. It is essential to consult a doctor or pharmacist before taking any medicines.

Barberry (Berberis vulgaris)

‣ **Side effects**: Barberry may induce stomach upset, nausea, and diarrhea in some people, especially if consumed in large quantities.

‣ **Contraindications**: Pregnant women are advised against

using barberry.

▸ **Interactions**: Barberry could interact with medications such as anticoagulants and blood pressure medications, potentially enhancing their effects. Consult your doctor before taking barberry to avoid adverse interactions.

Burdock (Arctium lappa)

▸ **Side effects**: Burdock root is generally considered safe, but it may cause stomach upset, diarrhea, or allergic skin reactions in some individuals.

▸ **Contraindications**: Caution should be exercised in people allergic to Asteraceae family plants (artichoke, marigold, daisy) and those with bile duct obstruction.

▸ **Interactions**: It may interact with diabetic medications and diuretics, so it is advisable to consult a doctor or pharmacist before combining it with medications.

Chamomile (Matricaria chamomilla)

▸ **Side effects**: These may include allergic reactions such as itching, skin rashes, or difficulty breathing, especially in individuals sensitive to the daisy family's plants.

▸ **Contraindications**: Avoid use during pregnancy, as it may cause uterine contractions, and in individuals with known allergies to plants of the Asteraceae family (marigold, daisy, artichoke, chicory).

▸ **Interactions**: Interactions may occur with medications such as anticoagulants, sedatives, and diabetes medications, potentially affecting their effects. Consult a doctor or pharmacist before combining chamomile with drugs.

Chicory (Cichorium intybus)

▸ **Side effects**: Chicory is generally safe for most individuals when consumed in average amounts as part of food. However, in high doses, it can lead to side effects like stomach upset, diarrhea, and skin irritation in some people.

‣ **Contraindications**: Individuals allergic to plants in the Asteraceae family, such as ragweed, daisy, and marigold, may find chicory unsuitable. Caution is advised for individuals with gallstones, as chicory could exacerbate the condition.

‣ **Interactions**: Due to its vitamin K content, Chicory may interact with specific medications, like blood thinners. It may also interact with diabetes medications, potentially lowering blood sugar levels.

Dandelion (Taraxacum officinale)

‣ **Side effects**: Although dandelion is generally considered safe for most individuals when consumed in average amounts through food, infusions, or supplements, some individuals may experience mild side effects such as stomach upset, diarrhea, or allergic skin reactions.

‣ **Contraindications**: Dandelion may not be suitable for some individuals, such as those with known allergies to plants in the Asteraceae family, like ragweed, marigold, and chamomile. Additionally, individuals with gallstones or stomach ulcers should avoid consuming dandelion without consulting a healthcare professional.

‣ **Interactions**: Dandelion may interact with certain drugs, such as diuretics, diabetes drugs, or blood thinners. If you take any medications, you must regularly talk to your doctor or pharmacist before taking dandelion.

Dong quai (Angelica sinensis)

‣ **Side effects**: Dong quai may cause sun sensitivity, increased blood pressure, diarrhea, skin rashes, and stomach upset in some individuals.

‣ **Contraindications**: Not recommended for use during pregnancy and lactation. It should also be avoided in people with bleeding disorders and those taking anticoagulants.

▸ **Interactions**: Dong quai may interact with drugs that affect blood clotting, such as anticoagulants and antiplatelet drugs. It may also interact with medications metabolized by the liver. It is recommended to consult a doctor or pharmacist before using dong quai if you are taking any medication.

Echinacea (Echinacea purpurea)

▸ **Side effects**: It may trigger allergic reactions in some individuals, as well as stomach upset, nausea, headache, and skin rash.

▸ **Contraindications**: This product should not be used by people with autoimmune diseases, immune system disorders, or allergies to the daisy family plants.

▸ **Interactions**: Potential interactions with immunosuppressive drugs, liver medications, and specific heart medications. It is advisable to consult with your doctor or pharmacist.

Fennel (Foeniculum vulgare)

▸ **Side effects**: Fennel is typically safe when consumed in average amounts through food. Nevertheless, some people may experience mild side effects, such as stomach upset, allergic skin reactions, or sun sensitivity.

▸ **Contraindications**: Fennel may not be suitable for everyone. Individuals allergic to plants of the Apiaceae family, such as celery, parsley, or carrots, may experience allergic reactions. Due to potential hormonal effects, pregnant or breastfeeding women should consult a doctor or pharmacist before consuming large quantities of fennel.

▸ **Interactions**: Specific medications, such as blood thinners or diabetes medications, may interact. It is recommended that you check with your doctor.

Ginger (Zingiber officinale)

▸ **Side effects**: High doses may lead to some individuals' heartburn, diarrhea, or gastrointestinal irritation.

‣ **Contraindications**: Avoid individuals taking anticoagulant drugs or those with gallstones.

‣ **Interactions**: Ginger may interact with anticoagulants, antiplatelet, and blood pressure medications. Please consult a doctor or pharmacist before combining it with drugs.

Green tea (Camellia sinensis)

‣ **Side effects**: It is generally safe when consumed in moderation, but some individuals may experience stomach irritation, insomnia, nervousness, headache, or palpitations.

‣ **Contraindications**: Caution should be exercised in people sensitive to caffeine, pregnant women, nursing mothers, and young children. Large-quantity consumption should also be avoided in individuals with thyroid problems or who are sensitive to stimulants.

‣ **Interactions**: Green tea may interact with blood-thinning medications, blood pressure medications, stimulant medicines, and some chemotherapy drugs. If you are taking any medications, consult your doctor or pharmacist before taking green tea.

Lavender (Lavandula angustifolia)

‣ **Side effects**: Lavender is generally safe when applied topically or inhaled, but it may cause skin irritation or allergic reactions in some individuals.

‣ **Contraindications**: Caution is advised for individuals with allergies to lavender or other plants of the Lamiaceae family (mint, rosemary, sage, thyme, basil). Additionally, pregnant women should avoid using it during the first trimester.

‣ **Interactions**: Lavender may interact with sedative, hypnotic, and antidepressant medications, potentially enhancing their effects. If you take any medications, consult a doctor or pharmacist before using lavender products.

Licorice (Glycyrrhiza glabra)

‣ **Side effects**: These can include fluid retention, high blood pressure, electrolyte imbalances, and, in rare cases, muscle weakness or heart problems due to glycyrrhizin in high doses.

‣ **Contraindications**: Include avoiding consumption in large quantities for prolonged periods, especially in individuals with high blood pressure, heart problems, kidney failure, pregnancy, and lactation. Caution should also be exercised in individuals with diabetes.

‣ **Interactions**: These may occur with medications such as diuretics, corticosteroids, antihypertensives, and heart failure medications, as licorice may potentiate or diminish the effects of these drugs. It is recommended that a doctor or pharmacist be consulted before combining licorice with medicines to avoid negative interactions.

Milk thistle (Silybum marianum)

‣ **Side effects**: It is generally considered safe, but in some cases, it may cause stomach upset, diarrhea, or allergic reactions in sensitive individuals.

‣ **Contraindications**: Milk thistle should be avoided by people allergic to plants in the Asteraceae family (chamomile, chicory, yarrow, etc.) and those with severe liver disease unless under the supervision of their doctor.

‣ **Interactions**: It may interact with certain medications used to treat diabetes, blood pressure, or those that affect the liver. If you are taking any medications, it is essential to consult a doctor or pharmacist before using milk thistle supplements.

Nettle (Urtica dioica)

‣ **Side effects**: Some individuals may experience stomach upset, diarrhea, and gastrointestinal irritation. In rare cases, it may cause allergic reactions, such as an itchy mouth, swelling of the throat, or difficulty breathing.

‣ **Contraindications**: Avoid consumption in large quantities or for prolonged periods, as it may lead to adverse effects in sensitive individuals. Use caution in individuals with kidney disorders, uncontrolled diabetes, and low blood pressure.

‣ **Interactions**: Interactions may occur with medications such as anticoagulants, antihypertensives, and diabetes medications, as the plant may interfere with their efficacy. Consult a doctor or pharmacist before taking nettle if you are on any medication.

Peppermint (Mentha)

‣ **Side effects** are generally mild and may include heartburn, skin irritation in sensitive individuals, and, in rare cases, allergic reactions such as rashes.

‣ **Contraindications**: Avoid use in infants and young children, as it may cause respiratory problems, and in individuals with acid reflux or chronic heartburn, as it may exacerbate these symptoms.

‣ **Interactions**: Peppermint may interact with medications such as proton pump inhibitors and some blood pressure medications, potentially affecting their absorption and efficacy. Consult a doctor or pharmacist before combining peppermint with medicines.

Rhodiola (Rhodiola rosea)

‣ **Side effects**: Rhodiola is generally well tolerated, but it may cause insomnia, irritability, dizziness, dry mouth, or increased blood pressure in some cases.

‣ **Contraindications**: Avoid use in people with bipolar disorder, schizophrenia, anxiety, or sleep disorders. Caution is also advised in pregnant or breast-feeding women.

‣ **Interactions**: Rhodiola may interact with medications for diabetes, hypertension, antidepressants, and stimulant medications. Please consult a doctor or pharmacist before combining it with other medicines.

Rosemary (Rosmarinus officinalis)

‣ **Side effects**: Rosemary is generally safe when used in average amounts, but may cause skin irritation or allergic reactions in some individuals.

‣ **Contraindications**: Avoid use in pregnant or breastfeeding women. Caution is also advised in individuals with allergies to other plants of the Lamiaceae family (mint, sage, thyme, basil, lavender).

‣ **Interactions**: Rosemary may interact with blood pressure medications, blood thinners, diabetes medications, and medications for thyroid problems. Please consult a doctor or pharmacist before combining it with other medicines.

Turmeric (Curcuma longa)

‣ **Side effects**: Stomach upset, heartburn, diarrhea, and skin allergies may occur in rare cases.

‣ **Contraindications**: Turmeric may not be suitable in large quantities for people with gallstones, bile duct obstruction, stomach ulcers, or known allergies to turmeric.

‣ **Interactions**: Turmeric may interact with medications such as anticoagulants, antiplatelet drugs, medications to reduce heartburn, and some diabetes drugs. It is advisable to check with your doctor or pharmacist.

Valerian (Valeriana officinalis)

‣ **Side effects**: Valerian is generally safe, but it may cause drowsiness, dizziness, dry mouth, headache, or upset stomach in some individuals.

‣ **Contraindications**: Avoid use in pregnant women, nursing mothers, young children, and individuals with liver disease.

Caution is also advised in individuals who drive or perform tasks requiring attention.

▸ **Interactions**: Valerian may interact with sedative drugs, antidepressants, anticonvulsants, and alcohol, enhancing their effects. Please consult a doctor or pharmacist before combining it with other medicines.

FINAL NOTE

Thank you very much for choosing this book to accompany you on your path to complete health. If you find the information, advice, or remedies I share here useful, would you do me a favor? Taking a moment to leave your review or rating (several stars would be greatly appreciated) is an incredible way to help me continue creating valuable content while also guiding others who, like you, are seeking to improve their health and well-being. Thank you so much for being part of this wellness community!

With gratitude,

Isabel

Important Note on Printing and Shipping:
All of my paperback books are printed and distributed exclusively by Amazon and its affiliated printing facilities. If you encounter any issues with print quality or delivery, please contact Amazon Customer Service directly for assistance.

As the author, I have no control over these processes, so I kindly request that your reviews focus solely on the content, remedies, or information within this work. Some readers leave negative ratings due to shipping or binding issues, unaware that these matters are, unfortunately, entirely beyond my control and ability to resolve. Thank you from the bottom of my heart for your understanding!

AUTHOR'S BOOKS

- **ACID REFLUX**. Foods, Supplements & Medicinal Plants
- **ALLERGIES**. Foods, Supplements & Herbs
- **ANXIETY**. Foods, Supplements & Herbs
- **ARTHRITIS**. Foods, Supplements & Medicinal Plants
- **CHOLESTEROL**. Foods, Supplements & Medicinal Plants
- **DIABETES**. Foods, Supplements & Herbs
- **CONSTIPATION**. Foods, Supplements & Herbs
- **FIBROMYALGIA**. Foods, Supplements & Medicinal Plants
- **GASTRITIS**. Foods, Supplements & Herbs
- **HEMORRHOIDS**. Foods, Supplements & Herbs
- **HYPERTENSION**. Foods, Supplements & Medicinal Plants
- **INSOMNIA**. Foods, Supplements & Herbs
- **MENOPAUSE**. Foods, Supplements & Medicinal Plants
- **OSTEOARTHRITIS**. Foods, Supplements & Herbs
- **SIBO**. Foods, Supplements & Medicinal Plants
- **VARICOSE VEINS**. Foods, Supplements & Herbs

Roots that Inspire: From Obstacles to New Horizons

Born in 1971 in Gáldar, Gran Canaria, Isabel grew up in an environment steeped in tradition and ancestral wisdom. Surrounded by the knowledge of her homeland, she learned from an early age to appreciate the healing power of medicinal plants, home remedies, and the importance of nutrition as foundations for nurturing both body and soul. This heritage, passed down through generations, shaped her childhood and sparked a deep passion for natural medicine–a passion that would eventually become the guiding force of her life.

The journey, however, was not without obstacles. In her youth, Isabel faced a period of profound difficulty: after her separation, she embraced the sole responsibility of raising her daughters. These were challenging times, with motherhood pushing her to her limits while simultaneously fueling her determination to persevere. Even during moments of uncertainty, she remained steadfast, drawing strength from her unwavering commitment to her values and her profound connection to natural health, which always served as her refuge and inspiration.

Rather than yielding to adversity, Isabel channeled it into a drive for learning and growth. She dedicated countless hours to studying books on medicinal plants, exploring new healing methods, and deepening her knowledge of natural remedies. Over the years, she pursued extensive training in naturopathy, nutrition, and complementary therapies, often sacrificing personal comforts to follow her passion. Her dedication not only provided for her family but also enabled her to profoundly impact the lives of those who sought her guidance. People came to trust her wisdom, turning to her for advice and support, and her efforts ignited transformations in countless lives.

A pivotal moment came in the 1990s when she made the

decision to professionalize her calling. She embarked on formal training as a naturopath and therapist specializing in alternative health practices. This step was transformative, opening new doors and broadening her ability to serve others. Her expertise, combined with her authentic desire to help, allowed her to support a growing community of people. Every story of healing and recovery deepened her sense of purpose, and she rebuilt her life around her mission to uplift others.

But Isabel's hunger for knowledge and her desire to inspire others extended beyond her immediate community. In 2017, she took a bold new step: she began to write with the aim of sharing her hard-earned experiences and knowledge on a larger scale. Her books, written in an accessible and heartfelt style, are both informative and empowering. They seamlessly blend practical advice, recipes, and natural health alternatives, inspiring readers to embrace healthier, more balanced lifestyles. Every page radiates her warmth and passion, inviting readers to find solutions for their well-being from within and aligning them to the wisdom of nature.

Today, Isabel's work resonates with countless individuals, especially those seeking to regain their health or reconnect with a more intentional way of living. Her story stands as a powerful reminder that even the greatest challenges can lead to profound purpose. Through resilience and perseverance, she has not only transformed her own life but also paved the way for others to rediscover their harmony with nature and with themselves. Her legacy serves as a celebration of living in balance with the natural world and honoring the deep, inherent connection between humanity and the Earth—a testament that obstacles can be the stepping stones to new horizons and an invitation to care for our body, mind, and planet with respect, awareness, and love.

BIBLIOGRAPHY & SCIENTIFIC STUDIES

1. "La Guía completa sobre SIBO y Tratamientos Naturales" - Dra. Sarah Ballantyne

2. "Digestive Health with Real Food" - Aglaée Jacob

3. "Healthy Gut, Healthy You" - Dr. Michael Ruscio

4. "El poder de las Plantas Medicinales" - Anne McIntyre

5. "Herbal Antibiotics" - Stephen Harrod Buhner

6. "The Good Gut: Taking Control of Your Weight, Your Mood, and Your Long-term Health" - Justin Sonnenburg and Erica Sonnenburg

7. "La digestión es la cuestión" - Giulia Enders

8. "Eat Dirt" - Dr. Josh Axe

9. "Gut and Psychology Syndrome" - Dr. Natasha Campbell-McBride

10. "The Complete Gut Health Cookbook" - Pete Evans and Helen Padarin

11. "The SIBO Solution" - Shivan Sarna

12. "SIBO Made Simple" - Phoebe Lapine

13. "El Gran Libro de las Plantas Medicinales" - Jorge D. Pamplona Roger

14. "Digestive Wellness" - Dr. Elizabeth Lipski

15. "The Microbiome Solution" - Dr. Robynne Chutkan

16. "Natural Solutions for Digestive Health" - Dr. Jillian Sarno Teta

17. "Restoring Your Digestive Health" - Dr. Jordan Rubin and Dr. Joseph Brasco

18. "The Plant Paradox" - Dr. Steven R. Gundry

19. "El Libro de la Medicina Natural" - Dr. Jorge Pérez-Calvo Soler

20. "The Herbal Medicine-Maker's Handbook" - James Green

SCIENTIFIC STUDIES
1. "Antibacterial and Antioxidant Activities of Origanum vulgare L. Essential Oil" - K. Khosravi, S. Mazandarani, M. Yaghmaei

2. "Oregano Essential Oil as a Bioactive Food Component: A Review" - M. V. Busatta, R. S. Vidal, A. S. Popiolski

3. "Aloe Vera: A Short Review" - M. Sahu, R. Das, S. Sahu

4. "Effects of Aloe vera on Gastrointestinal Motility and Inflammatory Mediators" - D. V. Patel, D. K. Shah, A. N. Patel

5. "Amylase: A Novel Therapy for Small Intestinal Bacterial Overgrowth" - J. H. Lee, H. J. Park, S. H. Kim

6. "The Role of Amylase in the Gastrointestinal Tract: A Review" - N. A. Smith, P. J. Smith

7. "Berberine: A Natural Compound with Antimicrobial Activity" - C. A. Imenshahidi, H. Hosseinzadeh

8. "Berberine as a Treatment for Gastrointestinal Disorders" - L. C. Zhang, Z. W. Zeng

9. "Bromelain: Biochemical and Pharmacological Properties" - M. Pavan, L. Jain, N. Shraddha

10. "The Role of Bromelain in the Treatment of Gastrointestinal Disorders" - A. Maurer

11. "Curcuma longa and Its Therapeutic Benefits in the Management of Small Intestinal Bacterial Overgrowth" - P. S. Hegarty, M. A. Barry

12. "Curcuma longa: Phytochemistry and Medicinal Properties" - J. Gupta, V. K. Singhal

13. "Curcumin and Its Potential Role in Gut Health" - A. Jurenka

14. "Therapeutic Roles of Curcumin: Lessons Learned from

Clinical Trials" - M. Heger

15. "Glutamine: Biochemistry and Physiological Role" - D. E. Wilmore

16. "The Role of Glutamine in Intestinal Health and Gut-Associated Lymphoid Tissue: A Review" - A. R. Lacey, M. Wilmore

17. "Iron and Its Role in Gut Microbiota Modulation" - N. L. Zimmermann

18. "The Effect of Iron on Gut Microbiota: A Review" - R. B. G. Britton

19. "Inulin-type Fructans: A Review on Their Modulatory Effects on Gut Microbiota" - C. Roberfroid

20. "The Role of Inulin in Gut Health and Its Potential in the Treatment of Small Intestinal Bacterial Overgrowth" - M. Kolida, G. R. Gibson

21. "Ginger as an Antimicrobial Agent in Gastrointestinal Disorders" - A. Ali, N. Blunden, Y. Tanira

22. "The Therapeutic Potential of Ginger in Gastrointestinal Disorders" - M. K. Tripathi, A. N. Goda

23. "Magnesium and Its Role in Gastrointestinal Health: A Review" - R. Quamme

24. "The Impact of Magnesium on Gut Microbiota and Gastrointestinal Health" - J. P. Galland

25. "N-Acetylcysteine: A Review of Its Role in Gut Health" - E. Samuni, S. Chaimoff

26. "The Therapeutic Potential of N-Acetylcysteine in Gastrointestinal Disorders" - M. S. Elbini Dhouib, A. J. McMahon

27. "Omega-3 Fatty Acids and Their Role in Modulating Gut Microbiota" - Y. Yang, J. Lu

28. "The Influence of Omega-3 Fatty Acids on Gastrointestinal Health" - W. Calder

29. "Papain: A Review of Its Digestive and Therapeutic Benefits" - B. Arnon, M. Zuckerman

30. "Papain and Its Potential Role in Gut Health" - R. S. Murthy, S. S. Bhatt

31. "Fructo-oligosaccharides: Prebiotic Effects and Gut Microbiota Modulation" - Y. Wang, M. J. Gibson

32. "Prebiotic FOS and Their Impact on Gut Health" - G. R. Gibson, M. B. Roberfroid

33. "Galacto-oligosaccharides and Their Role as Prebiotics in Gastrointestinal Health" - N. Rastall, S. Gibson

34. "The Effects of GOS on Gut Microbiota and Its Potential in SIBO Treatment" - A. L. Depeint, T. J. Macfarlane

35. "Probiotics in Human Health: A Review of Broad Spectrum Probiotics" - S. V. Thakur, R. P. Sinha

36. "The Role of Broad Spectrum Probiotics in the Management of Small Intestinal Bacterial Overgrowth" - J. A. Sanders, G. R. Gibson

37. "Selenium and Its Role in Gut Health: A Comprehensive Review" - L. Rayman

38. "Selenium in the Gastrointestinal Tract: Physiological Role and Therapeutic Potential" - K. H. Brown, R. J. Arthur

39. "Vitamin B12 and Its Impact on Gut Microbiota and Gastrointestinal Health" - A. Watanabe, H. Yabuta

40. "The Role of Vitamin B12 in Gastrointestinal Disorders and Gut Health" - M. Arocha, L. C. Kozyraki

41. "Vitamin C: Its Role in Modulating Gut Microbiota and Gastrointestinal Health" - C. Carr, B. Frei

42. "The Impact of Vitamin C on Gut Health and Its Potential Therapeutic Benefits" - S. A. Jacob, A. Sotoudeh

43. "Vitamin D and Its Role in Gastrointestinal Health: A Review" - P. J. Meeker, S. M. Seamans

44. "The Influence of Vitamin D on Gut Microbiota and Its Potential in SIBO Management" - M. J. Berridge, R. L. Packer

45. "Zinc and Gut Health: A Critical Review of Its Role and Benefits" - A. S. Prasad

46. "The Role of Zinc in Gastrointestinal Health and Its Potential in Treating SIBO" - L. Shankar, P. Prasad

47. "Chicory Root: Its Prebiotic Effects and Impact on Gut Microbiota" - D. F. Delzenne, Y. P. M. De Bie

48. "Achicoria: Beneficios en la Salud Intestinal y Potencial Terapéutico" - L. López-Molina, M. Navarro

49. "The Antimicrobial and Health Benefits of Berberis vulgaris (Agracejo)" - M. Ivanov, M. K. Ghosh

50. "Agracejo y su Potencial en Salud Intestinal: Una Revisión" - J. M. Ortiz, R. C. Ledesma

51. "Ashwagandha: A Review of Its Role in Gastrointestinal Health" - D. S. Raut, A. Rege

52. "Therapeutic Effects of Ashwagandha on Gut Microbiota and Intestinal Health" - S. S. Mir, M. M. Al-Baradie

53. "Bacopa monnieri: A Review of Its Potential Benefits in Gastrointestinal Health" - C. Stough, J. P. Downey

54. "The Impact of Bacopa on Gut Microbiota and Its Potential in SIBO Management" - R. Walker, A. L. Silberstein

55. "Burdock (Bardana) Root: Health Benefits and Its Role in Gut Health" - H. Lin, M. Yang

56. "Bardana: Propiedades Antimicrobianas y Potencial en Salud Intestinal" - Y. S. Kim, J. Y. Lee

57. "Milk Thistle (Cardo Mariano): A Review of Its Gastrointestinal Benefits" - A. M. Haddad, N. S. Noor

58. "The Therapeutic Potential of Milk Thistle in Gastrointestinal Disorders" - J. Kroll, L. Shaw

59. "Dandelion (Diente de león): Antimicrobial Properties and Gut Health Benefits" - C. E. Schütz, E. R. Carle

60. "The Impact of Dandelion on Gut Health and Its Potential Therapeutic Uses" - L. Hu, G. Zhang

61. "Angelica sinensis (Dong quai): Its Role in Modulating Gut Microbiota" - H. Sun, X. Xue

62. "The Health Benefits of Dong Quai in Gastrointestinal Disorders" - J. Y. Zhou, Y. F. Zhang

63. "Echinacea and Its Role in Gastrointestinal Health: A Review" - M. S. Perry, R. H. Foster

64. "The Potential Benefits of Echinacea in Modulating Gut Microbiota" - H. Hudson, S. P. Vimalanathan

65. "Ginseng and Its Gastrointestinal Health Benefits: A Review" - S. K. Kim, H. S. Park

66. "The Role of Ginseng in Modulating Gut Microbiota and Its Potential in SIBO" - J. Y. Kang, S. J. Lee

67. "Fennel (Hinojo): Its Gastrointestinal Benefits and Antimicrobial Properties" - D. G. Srivastava, R. K. Kapoor

68. "The Impact of Fennel on Gut Health and Its Therapeutic Potential" - A. S. Badgujar, V. M. Jain

69. "Lavender and Its Role in Gastrointestinal Health: A Comprehensive Review" - N. Lis-Balchin, S. Hart

70. "The Therapeutic Potential of Lavender in Modulating Gut Microbiota" - E. Cavanagh, J. Wilkinson

71. "Chamomile (Manzanilla): Health Benefits and Its Role in Gut Health" - S. Srivastava, E. Shankar

72. "The Effects of Chamomile on Gastrointestinal Disorders and Microbiota" - M. McKay, J. B. Blumberg

73. "Peppermint (Menta) Oil: Gastrointestinal Benefits and Antimicrobial Effects" - A. Kligler, J. Chaudhary

74. "The Role of Peppermint in Modulating Gut Microbiota and Its Potential in SIBO" - S. Cash, A. Epstein

75. "Nettle (Ortiga): Its Antimicrobial Properties and Gastrointestinal Benefits" - F. Chrubasik, B. Roufogalis

76. "The Therapeutic Potential of Nettle in Gut Health and SIBO

Management" - A. E. Upton, M. J. Brain

77. "Licorice (Regaliz) and Its Role in Gastrointestinal Health: A Review" - R. A. Asl, H. Hosseinzadeh

78. "The Health Benefits of Licorice in Modulating Gut Microbiota" - S. M. Fiore, F. Eisenhut

79. "Rhodiola: Its Gastrointestinal Benefits and Potential Antimicrobial Effects" - V. Kucinskaite, J. Briedis

80. "The Role of Rhodiola in Modulating Gut Microbiota and SIBO Treatment" - S. Panossian, G. Wikman

81. "Rosemary and Its Impact on Gut Health: A Comprehensive Review" - M. E. López-Jiménez, J. A. Gómez-Plaza

82. "The Antimicrobial and Gastrointestinal Benefits of Rosemary" - A. Bozin, N. Mimica-Dukic

83. "Green Tea (Té verde): Its Role in Modulating Gut Microbiota and Gastrointestinal Health" - D. S. Yang, C. W. Lee

84. "The Therapeutic Potential of Green Tea in SIBO Management" - M. Cabrera, R. Artacho

85. "Valerian: Its Effects on Gut Health and Potential Antimicrobial Properties" - M. Peroutka, T. Schulz

86. "The Role of Valerian in Modulating Gastrointestinal Disorders" - B. M. Miyasaka, L. C. Atallah

FOODS THAT TRANSFORM

JUICES AND SMOOTHIES